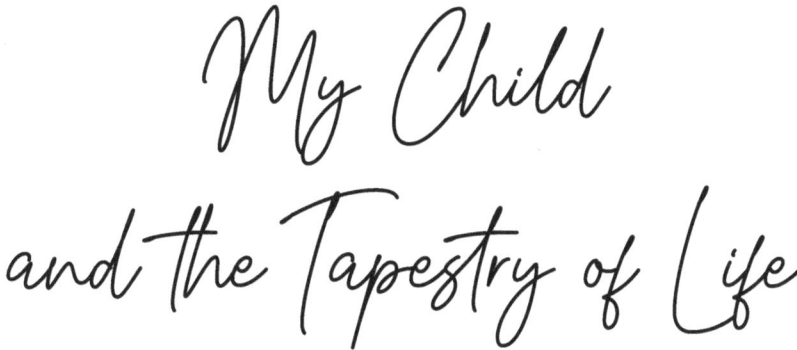

A Woman's Journey
to Heal the Little Girl Inside

written by
Megan Reda

My Child and the Tapestry of Life: An Autobiography

Copyright © 2020 Megan Reda

This book is copyright. Apart from any use permitted under *The Copyright Act 1968*, no part may be reproduced by any process without prior written permission from the publisher.

ISBN: 978-0-6488386-0-9 (print)
ISBN: 978-0-6488386-1-6 (ePub)

Self-published 2020 Megan Reda ©

All Bible Scriptures contained in this book are from the NKJV translation.

Scriptures marked NKJV are taken from the NEW KING JAMES VERSION (NKJV): Scripture taken from the NEW KING JAMES VERSION®. Copyright © 1982 by Thomas Nelson, Inc. Used by permission. All rights reserved.

Edited by Hayley Ward
Cover design by Candice Jade Graphics
Photography by Shazza J Photography
Typesetting: Chris Moore
Model (front and back cover) Megan Hyland
Administrator: Jacquie Hyland

Contact me at *Heart Weaves* for any further discussions of any topics found within this book at www.meganreda.com and also download my Mental Health, Spiritual Awakening, Trauma Healing and Wellness FREE PDF workbook.

*Whatever battle or struggle you are facing,
whatever dream you are pursuing,
with faith, hope and love,
you can have the VICTORY!*

Megan Reda

Foreword

It's not very often in life you meet someone you instantly connect with; you don't know why, but there's a deeper meaning to this instant friendship. The more you get to know the person you realise that you have a similar story or life journey. This was true when I met Megan. It was like finding a long-lost friend.

As our friendship grew over time, through talking, sharing and many cups of tea, I got to know what a beautiful, honest and compassionate woman she is. When Megan told me she'd written a book about her life; naturally, I was curious and excited to read it. I had the honour of being able to read the draft copy of this book, in which Megan so bravely shares her story.

This book details Megan's encounters through deep, painful trauma and mental health. She then shares her incredible experience of how with the power of belief and faith, she began to heal. This was when I realised the deep connection I had to Megan. It was because I had experienced traumas and battles with mental health throughout childhood and into adulthood.

If you or someone you know has been through trauma or mental health issues, her story will give you hope that healing is also possible for you.

Through Megan's dedication and devotion, it took over two decades to write this book as her healings unfolded. Told with pure honesty and heart, this is an inspiring story that tells one woman's incredible journey from deep despair, then to finding faith and the courage to begin an existence full of love, peace and the strength to live her best life.

Megan's story has helped guide me on my continued healing path. I wish the same for you – the reader.

Thank you, Megan, for sharing your story.

Love and Gratitude,

Laura Ray

Educator. Business owner.

Acknowledgements

It's too difficult to mention the many, many people I would like to thank for their love, support and contributions to my life.

However, I would like to acknowledge the generosity and inspirations of my adopted mother for her unconditional love and hours of tears and laughter during this process—my dear lifelong friend Libby for her years of friendship, standing by me and being there for me through the hard times. To my beautiful friend Laura for always cheering me on and being such a positive light in my life. Also, Jill, for her insightful prayer support needed to birth this vision, Candice for her patience and beautiful design skills, Sharon for her talent behind the camera, and the IT expertise from Jacquie for guiding me in the final processes of bringing this book into reality.

To my dear friends who read draft copies and gave me feedback, I value you.

For the time spent sharing my journey with you all to bring me to this point, I say thank you.

The Weaver

My life is but a weaving
between my God and me.
I cannot choose the colours
He weaveth steadily.
Oft' times He weaveth sorrow;
and I in foolish pride
forget He sees the upper,
and I the underside.
Not 'til the loom is silent
and the shuttles cease to fly,
will God unroll the canvas,
and reveal the reason why.
The dark threads are as needful
in the weaver's skilful hand,
as the threads of gold and silver
in the pattern, He has planned.
He knows, He loves, He cares;
nothing this truth can dim.
He gives the very best to those
Who leave the choice to Him.

Grant Colfax Tullar

This book is lovingly dedicated to

My birth mother and father
My adopted mother and father
My three beautiful children

All the people in my life who have
woven their lives into mine, and
given me a story to tell.

Table of Contents

INTRODUCTION – *A Stitch in Time* 1

CHAPTER 1 – *My Beginning* 3
CHAPTER 2 – *A New Pattern* 16
CHAPTER 3 – *Childhood Days* 27
CHAPTER 4 – *My Friend Jacky* 44
CHAPTER 5 – *Hello Supernatural* 47
CHAPTER 6 – *Desperate for Love* 55
CHAPTER 7 – *Unforetold Future* 63
CHAPTER 8 – *Is Someone Looking out for Me?* 67
CHAPTER 9 – *Overflowing with Charisma* 70
CHAPTER 10 – *Just for a Giggle* 80
CHAPTER 11 – *Born to Charm* 89
CHAPTER 12 – *Divine Appointment* 98
CHAPTER 13 – *A Brand New Life* 111
CHAPTER 14 – *The Devil Himself* 118
CHAPTER 15 – *Filled with Fire* 123
CHAPTER 16 – *What? Alan's Return* 125

CHAPTER 17 – *The Wardrobe Door* 128

CHAPTER 18 – *It wasn't His Time* 130

CHAPTER 19 – *The Accident* 133

CHAPTER 20 – *Following the Leader* 138

CHAPTER 21 – *Psalm 23* 150

CHAPTER 22 – *A Dark Valley* 154

CHAPTER 23 – *The Shadow of Death* 159

CHAPTER 24 – *My Angels of Escape* 163

CHAPTER 25 – *The Day I met my Mother* 175

CHAPTER 26 – *The Day I met my Father* 184

CHAPTER 27 – *Life After Alan* 189

CHAPTER 28 – *Cries from Hell* 205

CHAPTER 29 – *I will Find my Way* 207

CHAPTER 30 – *The Loss of a Loved One* 212

CHAPTER 31 – *Wardrobe Door – You are Defeated* 214

CHAPTER 32 – *Thank you for Saying Goodbye* 223

CHAPTER 33 – *Unfinished Business* 225

CHAPTER 34 – *Completely Healed* 229

CHAPTER 35 – *Breath of Heaven* 231

INTRODUCTION

A Stitch in Time

I have heard it said that in every person's life there is a book.

Here is mine.

It might sound cliché, *but I was born to write this book.* As each chapter weaves threads together, eventually, you will see why I make such a bold statement.

I say weave because my life – if I may use the analogy – is like an intricate, embroidered tapestry. While some threads appear dull, others are incredibly vibrant, and some strands are an unfortunate black. Some threads stitch with ease while others get knotted, frayed, and pulled. Since I was a little girl, I started stitching these seemingly insignificant threads onto the everyday fabric of my life, and over time, they now form a very startling picture.

My story is one of complete transparency, universal destiny, and many times, the unbelievable! I only ask that you have an open heart and mind as I share my journey.

ALL names and some places have been changed out of respect and privacy of the people involved.

The first two chapters take place before I, Emma Morgan, was born. While they read like fiction, these chapters, like the rest of my story, are factual events to the best of my knowledge.

As you read *My Child and the Tapestry of Life* you may find the story identifies with your life, someone you know, or even your child.

It is my deepest desire that my story will bring you hope, encouragement, and healing for your journey.

I have the utmost respect for whatever belief or religion you have or don't have. This book is not about judgement. Rather, it is about sharing my experiences of a realm I was thrust into, which exposed me to a beautiful, incredible force that is far greater than anything I have ever experienced here on earth.

As I acknowledged it and surrendered, amazing things happened that were beyond my human capabilities, knowledge, and understanding. And because of it, I have learned with faith, hope, and love – ANYTHING is possible.

I invite you now, dear reader, to come with me on my journey as I reveal to you, stitch by stitch, the design of my life.

CHAPTER 1

My Beginning

"**P**ush, Laurie! That's a girl! *Push*, keep it going. Keep pushing. Keep pushing, almost there, that's it, and relax!" Nurse Jacobs wiped Laurie's forehead with a damp cloth and, in a calm but direct voice said, "Your baby's head has crowned. This next contraction, you will need to use all your strength – just one more *big* push when I tell you." "I can't," Laurie said, utterly exhausted. "I can't do it anymore!"

Her body was wet and clammy with sweat, and the sheets on the delivery bed were saturated.

"You can." Nurse Jacobs was firm. "Your baby is nearly here, and it's almost over." Laurie winced as another contraction began. "When I say push, push with everything you have." Nurse Jacobs waited a moment. She took Laurie's hand and held it tightly. "Okay, here we go," Nurse Jacobs said, entirely focused, "breathe, breathe, breathe. Here we go, Laurie! Now, *PUSH!*"

Laurie took a huge breath and gave it her all. The pain was excruciating. Every nerve ending in her body exploded as she screwed up her face in sheer determination.

The whole area between her legs was stretching wider, and the pain burned like fire. Her lower body felt like it was tearing in two. Suddenly, a warm flow released the intense pressure, and Nurse Jacobs praised her for a job well done. Laurie lay numb and exhausted.

After many laboured hours, sounds of relief now filled the birthing ward. *Her baby was born.*

Nurse Jacobs' demeanour instantly changed as she spoke with suppressed emotion. Her words were matter of fact and without warmth

– even a slight sadness in her tone. "It's a girl. Laurie, you have just given birth to a little girl."

Laurie lay fatigued on the sweaty hospital mattress. Her head and chest pounded. Full of anxiety and sore all over, Laurie lay still as she listened to the high-pitched cry of her newborn baby. The desperate call penetrated right through her and pierced her heart. It sounded as though her baby was hurt. *What are those nurses doing to my baby to cause her so much distress?* She had an all-consuming desire to reach out and take her baby in her arms. To see and feel her well-deserved reward for enduring the past nine months.

But Nurse Jacobs – matronly and solemn – was in charge. She took the baby in her arms and walked straight over to the scales. Synchronising with the other nurses, like a well-rehearsed play they had performed many times before, the baby was weighed, measured, and checked all over. Their routine was smooth and professional as they moved to a tune of hushed whispers.

Everything appeared normal – although the baby would not stop crying.

Laurie, worried something was wrong, asked, "Is she all right?"

"Yes, she's perfect," chirped one of the nurses. "She's got ten fingers and ten toes, a mop of brown hair, and she is exactly six pounds."

Nurse Jacobs quickly turned and glared at the nurse as if she was saying too much, and the nurse promptly looked down in obedience and went back to sorting the soiled linen. Laurie's baby continued to cry frantically, and there was nothing she could do.

It was now apparent to Nurse Jacobs that there was something unusual about this baby's cry. She waved to the nurses to hurry up with their routine checks, hoping the baby would feel secure wrapped tightly in a blanket – the last step of the process.

Laurie couldn't block out her baby's penetrating sound, so she whispered to herself, "Don't cry, my little one, don't cry!" *Little one* was the pet name she had called her baby.

One of the other nurses heard Laurie's mutterings and quietly went over to her and asked, "What did you say, Laurie? Did you want to see your baby?"

Nurse Jacobs quickly turned again, shaking her head. She glared at the nurse to be quiet. Laurie set her head aside as a tear trickled from her eye. She rolled over, trying to be resilient, and desperately trying not to cry. Laurie knew this day would come. She knew it would be hard. But not *this* hard.

Every maternal instinct inside her was screaming to reach out and hold her baby close to her.

But she knew that if she looked at her little girl, just a glance, she could never let her go. Now her baby had been born, she wanted her more than ever. But this was not to be. She had to allow these nurses to take her child away from her – forever.

Laurie was angry at God and full of hate. She hated her parents; and Doug, the baby's father. She hated Dr Bray, their family doctor, and she hated these nurses.

With a cold heart, Laurie replied rudely to the nurse, "No, I don't want to see her!"

Laurie gripped the sheets so tightly her fingers began to sting. She tried not to flip into an uncontrollable panic as she was, at this very moment, separated from her baby, and there was nothing she could do. Laurie felt sick. She wanted to vomit. The sound of her baby girl crying was tormenting.

Laurie whispered to herself again, "Hush now, little one. Don't cry. Hush now."

This self-soothing was to comfort herself more than anything. Laurie's eyes burned with sadness. Her heart ached with hopelessness. Merely taking a breath was painful. She was trying hard not to hyperventilate and forced herself to concentrate on deep, slow breaths.

As Laurie lay in turmoil, she became aware that a nurse had taken her baby out of the delivery room. The once piercing cry was now distant, and Laurie clung to the fading shrill until there was no sound. Tears welled up in her eyes. It was at that moment she was internally broken.

A tangible, dark grief hovered above Laurie, and without invitation, settled upon her.

Eventually, a nurse came to shower Laurie and took her to a hospital bed for some rest. It was a four-bed ward occupied by three other women who already had their babies. Laurie made her grand entrance as the nurse pushed her through the doorway in a wheelchair. As soon as Laurie saw the three women, shame flooded her. Her arms were empty. Two of them were breastfeeding, while another proudly held her obvious prize. The women looked at her, wide-eyed and keen to share more newly born excitement.

One of them asked, "What did you have?"

Laurie, unprepared for such a question, blurted out without thinking, "I… I lost my baby."

There was an awkward silence. Laurie, infused with anger, hated that woman for even asking. *Why had they brought her into a ward full of mothers with their newborns when she had nothing? How could the nurses be so cruel to her?*

Quietly, Laurie slunk into the bed and rolled over to get some much-needed rest. She tried to block out where she was. Even though her body lay still from exhaustion, she couldn't stop her mind racing back over her life and how it had led her to here. Her thoughts took her back to her childhood.

Her parents, Henry and Mavis Patterson, married in 1943. Mavis was born in Australia and endured a strict upbringing throughout the Depression years. She was often ill with asthma, and her childhood, alongside her sister, was tough. Mavis's mother had married at a very early age and found it hard to cope. One day her mother decided that she couldn't look after her two girls anymore and walked out on the family. Mavis was only five years old at the time. Her father remarried, and her stepmother never accepted either of them.

Henry's family, on the other hand, migrated to Australia from England when he was six years old. They lived life very plainly, and Henry and his brother had a good relationship. In later years, Henry's brother played the Hawaiian guitar, so they formed a band and subsequently performed on the radio several times. Henry became a butcher, married Mavis, and they bought a local butcher business. They worked long hours and provided an excellent service to the community.

Laurie had other siblings, Colin, an older brother, Robert, a younger brother, who had sadly passed away, and Lucy, who was fourteen years younger than herself. Her mother, Mavis, called Laurie the black sheep of the family, which only added fuel to the fire concerning her insecurities and rebellious attitude.

A never-mentioned family tragedy a decade ago had driven a wedge between Laurie and her mother. It was this suppressed, *let's sweep it under the carpet* attitude, that altered Laurie's dynamic in the home.

When Laurie was eight years old her duty was to babysit her younger brother, Robert. On this particular day, Robert had been asleep in his cot for a long time, and Laurie thought how easy this had been for her. She didn't even have to give him a bottle or tend to him at all.

Later, Mavis returned home and checked on Robert to find he had died in his sleep. His bowel had twisted and it was this unknown medical condition that had silently taken his life. Laurie inwardly blamed herself, reading her mother's grief as direct anger towards her. This shaped Laurie's defiance and rebellion. The incident was never spoken of again, and everyone seemed to – get on with life – but Laurie never could. It was at this point she started to crave love and acceptance. She desired a boyfriend, although her self-esteem was extremely low.

Laurie was five-foot-ten – tall for 18 – and she hated the fact that she always towered over everybody. Black shoulder-length hair framed her face, and her small, dark eyes absorbed every detail of the life around her. Having braces on her teeth didn't help her self-confidence. A deep thinker and socially awkward, she didn't fit in, either at school or at home.

Meeting Doug had given her hope for a happy future. Douglas Williams was a 24-year-old Scot. Tanned, handsome, and charismatic, he moved with natural, athletic grace. Every girl was captivated by his hypnotic blue eyes. And one day, he just happened to glance at Laurie.

It all happened very quickly. Laurie had wandered down to the neighbourhood oval to watch the local boys play football. Her attention was drawn to him immediately, and he looked over at her. Their eyes made instant contact, and her stomach fluttered like a thousand butterflies. No one had ever looked at her that way. She giggled and smiled, extending a silent invitation for him to approach her, and hoped that it would be enough for him to do so after the game.

It was the most exciting moment of her life.

Laurie never lived by the house rules as she had an iron will and a thunderous spirit. She did whatever she wanted to do, even if that meant blotting out all sense of her morals and responsible behaviour. And right now, she wanted romance.

Incredibly shy and with no confidence in her appearance, Laurie was easy prey when Doug's sparkling blue eyes met hers. Now the game had finished and – just as she'd hoped – he walked over to her.

"Would you like a ride home?" Doug asked smoothly.

His voice was silky and captivating. Laurie's chest pounded – she froze, and nodded, concentrating on smiling without showing her teeth. It didn't take much to be smitten; a look, a smile, and an invitation to drive her home. And maybe the fact that he had a car.

"Well, you'd better tell me where you live," Doug said with a smirk.

"Okay," Laurie answered softly.

One word was all she could manage. Besides a brief introduction, there was no conversation on the drive home. Laurie was so shy and didn't know what to say.

"Just pull over there, in front of *that* shop," Laurie said, pointing her finger and a little embarrassed.

"Your dad owns a butcher shop?" Doug asked.

"Yes. It's the family business," Laurie told him.

What a stupid thing to say, she thought. But Doug smiled.

"Come over here, next to me. Are you cold?" He asked.

She wasn't, but she replied, "Yes."

Doug kissed her. Laurie was so embarrassed, ashamed of the harsh metal in her mouth. His hands wandered quickly, and before too long; they were both in the back seat. That night, in Doug's car, in front of her family home and their respectable butcher business, she gave him more than a goodnight kiss. Laurie knew it was wrong, but Doug was very persistent, and after his crooning, sweet affections she gave in. Laurie believed it was the start of something beautiful, but she never heard from him again. He had used her, and she was ashamed and broken-hearted.

It was a couple of months later when Laurie suspected she might be pregnant. They had only done *it* once, but once was enough. She knew she had to find Doug and let him know.

Perhaps he would do the right thing and offer to marry her?

So, once again, Laurie walked to the neighbourhood oval, and after their game, awkwardly approached Doug with the news. She hadn't seen him for a long while and felt sick with nerves. Laurie told him her plight, and he hinted at the possibility that it might not be his. She knew it was. There had been no one else, but there was no way he was going to marry her. He was a very busy boy, giving many of the other local girls a ride home as well. Doug said he had money and could take care of it, meaning – abort the baby. Put on the spot, Laurie didn't know how to reply. She just shook her head. Doug dismissed her quickly, and from that moment on, he acted as if they never met.

Laurie was devastated, abandoned and alone. She knew she'd have to tell her father and mother eventually but held off for as long as she could. She knew how this could impact the family and their business. They had worked hard to establish their butcher shop, and they were very proud of it.

Laurie's belly started to poke out, and she knew she couldn't keep it a secret any longer.

Shamefully, she told her mother. Mavis was shocked beyond belief, angry, and disappointed. Laurie had shattered any respect her mother had for her. Now, Laurie was nothing but a tart in her mother's eyes. A label she would wear for the rest of her life.

Mavis erupted. "Well, having it is one thing, but keeping it is another! You are going to have to put this baby up for adoption!"

Laurie shouted back, "Don't you think I already know that! Anyway, I wouldn't want my baby to be anywhere near *him!*"

She was referring to her father. Henry was a strict man, and at times Laurie thought him very unfair and mean. They clashed terribly, mainly because they shared the same strong-willed personality.

Laurie continued shouting at her mother, "He would delight in destroying the soul of my baby, just like he has destroyed mine!"

"Stop being so dramatic, Laurie. And stop being disrespectful," Mavis retaliated. "Your father is the head of this house, and he always does what is best for us!"

"What, like drinking every night and making a fool of himself?" Laurie shouted again.

"Stop that, Laurie! Stop that at once!" Mavis snapped back, defending her husband. "He works hard to provide for all of us. Don't you forget that!"

Laurie wasn't going to listen to her mother anymore. They could argue for hours. She stormed out the front door, letting it crash behind her.

"Where are you going?" Mavis questioned her.

Laurie shouted back. "Anywhere to get away from *you!*"

She stood at the end of the veranda and lit a cigarette. She wasn't going to give up smoking throughout her pregnancy, even though there was a growing awareness that it was terrible for the baby. Tobacco was the only thing that calmed her nerves.

Mavis called out, "Well, don't come back until your father has had his dinner! And I'll give him a few more drinks, so he's numb before he's landed with your news! Your promiscuity is going to devastate him.

God forbid anyone ever finding out! You will have to go and stay with Aunt Gretta until it's all over, and I will ring Dr Bray straight away. You'd better not be the ruin of us and our business!"

Laurie didn't retaliate. All they cared about was their precious business. She would be happy to move away. She loved Aunt Gretta. More than she loved them.

The year was 1961. An unforgivable shame and stigma haunted any girl falling pregnant out of wedlock. Families were shunned in their neighbourhoods, ignored politely at church, and the government offered no financial support.

Later that evening, Henry was on the warpath. He was drunk and angry. His voice boomed throughout the house.

"*LAURIE!* Come here, you harlot! You are a disgrace to this family!"

Petrified of her father, Laurie ran to her bedroom for safety. She placed the back of a chair under the doorknob in an attempt to ward him off, but he found her and kept shouting obscenities at her through the door.

Luckily, Mavis *had* given him more to drink, and eventually, Henry gave up and slumped in his armchair, until he fell asleep. From then on, Laurie strategically planned her every move to keep out of her father's way.

Filled with anxiety about having the baby, Laurie would have done anything to end her deep sadness. She took a knife from her father's butcher shop to cut her wrists but was unsuccessful. Her mother, wondering why the bathroom door was locked, demanded that Laurie open it, only to find her covered in blood from wounds on her wrists. Mavis intervened just in time, applying pressure and then bandages. Laurie spent the rest of the day recovering in bed, and as it was cold enough for long sleeves, no one besides her mother ever knew what she had attempted to do.

A month later, still deeply depressed, Laurie took one of her mother's knitting needles into the shower and tried to abort the baby herself. Blood ran down the inside of her legs as she watched red water wash away down the plughole. But the baby remained inside her! Another failed attempt to end her misery. Laurie resolved herself to the fact that there was no option left but to have this child.

Almost four months along and with adoption as her only choice, Laurie needed one more thing from Doug: his signature on the legal paperwork. She plucked up enough courage and walked down to the oval one evening to see him after footy training. Doug was shocked to see her but signed the adoption papers as quickly as he could with the hope of having nothing more to do with her.

As her mother had promised, the day arrived for Laurie to go and stay with Aunt Gretta. Laurie was relieved. Aunt Gretta was her favourite. A quiet and gentle soul with a simple faith in God, Gretta looked past Laurie's actions and treated her with love and kindness.

"Here, Laurie, drink this." Gretta's voice was soothing as she handed Laurie a mug. "Warm milk and honey are good for you and the baby."

"Thank you, Aunty," Laurie said, appreciatively.

"And come over here next to me." Gretta patted the cushion on an outdoor chair. "Sit with your back to the sun. It is like medicine!"

Gretta prayed regularly over the baby in Laurie's tummy and spoke healing words to the little forming life. As she gently laid her hand on Laurie's stomach, Gretta said, "You know sweet child, our lives are like a tapestry. God is the master weaver, and He is always busy at work. There are times in our life; we only see the back, which is a mess of pulled threads, frayed ends, and painful knots. What we don't understand is that God knows what He is doing! If you trust in Him, it will all work out. On the other side, He is creating a beautiful picture you will eventually see. *In His way, and in His time.*"

Laurie couldn't see *how* God could make a beautiful picture out of the mess she was in, but she felt a peace at her Aunt's house she had never felt before. Laurie used to pretend Aunt Gretta was her mother, though she couldn't live in her pretend world forever. Her reality was alive and growing steadily.

Once a month, Laurie went home for a visit, but it was far from a loving reunion. The car ride there and back was the only beautiful part of the experience. As Gretta's car pulled up outside the family home, Mavis would be waiting with a white bed sheet in her hands. 'Sheet Day,' as Laurie used to call it. Her mother would walk briskly to the car and cover Laurie with the cumbersome cloth – from head to toe – hiding her identity and concealing her shame. It was incredibly stuffy, and Laurie couldn't see where she was going as Mavis scurried her into the house and out of sight.

The sheet routine was just as suffocating as the unloving welcome she always received from her drunk and abusive father. He was angry because she came home every month with her ever-growing belly. Protecting his butcher business was his only concern. Granted, if anyone saw Laurie *knocked up*, as he called it, tongues would wag, and indeed their reputation scarred for life. It would be a certainty; they would lose all of their customers.

As soon as Laurie stepped inside the house, Henry's jeers towards her were continuous, and his alcohol-soaked words slurred with vengeful spite. Mavis did her best to keep him calm, but Henry hunted Laurie down like prey and hissed his disgust like a snake.

"Where are you? You are a disgrace to this family, Laurie! You and your harlot ways! You have no idea the calamity you have brought on this family. *AND*, God forbid this business!"

"Such a calamity!" he'd shout. Henry's eyes were wild and bloodshot. He'd work himself into such a rage, staggering around the house trying to find her, that he foamed at the mouth like a rabid dog. Every visit was the same. She hated her father.

Laurie's bedroom was not a safe place to hide anymore, so her only escape was to climb inside a musty, old, brown wooden wardrobe in the spare room where her father kept his winter coats. It reeked of mothballs and stale cigarettes, but with the door open – just a crack – she was able to get some fresh air and keep a lookout. For some reason, he never came into this room.

Although Laurie was well hidden, she panicked at the sound of her father's heavy footsteps drawing closer to her hiding place. She felt sick, and the baby kicked wildly inside her, sensing her anxiety and fear.

Laurie's whole body would shake inside the wardrobe. The stale, musty smell overpowered her, and she felt sick to her stomach. She gasped for air through the crack of the wardrobe door and tried to breathe slowly and deeply as her fear consumed her.

Aware that her baby was reacting to her trauma, she would rub her belly and whisper, "It's all right, my little one. I know you don't like it in this wardrobe – nor do I – but we're safe here," and she continued to stroke her stomach in an attempt to soothe her baby's distress.

But, unbeknown to her, Laurie's anxieties pulsed deep into the fabric and DNA of her baby.

Laurie's fear spewed out a substance so vile, it permeated through the protective amniotic fluid and rooted itself into the baby's memory cells. The baby couldn't help but absorb it. The toxic, anxious substance imprinted a voice into the growing fabric of this child.

It said, *"I am in you, and around you. My essence is fear! You will never escape me. You will only see life through my perceptions of dread! You will be anxious about the day and the night! Do you hear me? I am evil. I will bring torment into your life. You will try to cover up my pain with anything you can find to shut me out, but you will never escape me. Be afraid, child. Be very afraid of everyone and everything. As dark as this wardrobe is, like a shadow of death, I will hover over you and be waiting for you around every corner throughout your life! Do you understand? Every breath you take will be one of fear! My toxic substance is so deep inside you, and there is no escape."*

CLANG! The sudden sound of the hospital meal trolley wobbling inside the room brought Laurie's thoughts back to the present. Her lunch had arrived. She wasn't hungry, but she sat up anyway. Day after day, Laurie had no visitors, no flowers, no wishes of celebration or condolence.

The day before Laurie was due to go home, she asked if she could leave the hospital for a short time to sit in the park across the road. Her request was met with sympathy by the staff, and she was permitted to do so.

The park was so peaceful. All the flowers were in full bloom, and the green grass was as smooth as velvet. Ducks swam freely on the lake. The air was chilly, though a touch of sunshine reflected silver glitters on the water. Laurie sat, aching in her grief. For a long while, she stared blankly out over the water. She blamed God for taking her baby away from her, but finally, in desperation, she whispered a prayer, "God, I put my baby in your hands. Please, take care of her."

Tears welled up in her eyes. She covered her face with both her hands and started crying.

"Please forgive me, my little one. Someday I hope I will see you again. Until then, I will keep you in my heart, and I will never forget you. You are, and always will be, my child."

CHAPTER 2

A New Pattern

Gina sat patiently in Dr Bray's waiting room. Looking around, she noticed there wasn't an empty chair. Dr Bray had a good reputation, and many people, even from the outer suburbs, came for his expertise and kind manner. He was well-respected in the community, and for good reason. He always went above and beyond in caring for his patients.

Gina had sat on these chairs many times. Falling pregnant with her first child, Graham had been difficult, but now, trying for a second child was an impossibility. Conceiving wasn't a problem; keeping the baby inside her womb was. For four years, every conception had ended in miscarriage. Gina, worn out and heartbroken, needed help.

As she expected a lengthy wait, Gina sat quietly and closed her eyes. The morning sun filtered through the window, and the warmth made her feel very relaxed, almost sleepy. She reflected on memories of her own life growing up.

"Gina, if anyone asks, tell them you are going to work in an office." This advice came during a conversation she had one day with her darling mother, Florence James. Gina had straight brown hair, blue eyes, and a slim frame. Working in an office sounded all right if she thought about it at all. But at 12 years of age, the beckoning call of the river was far more urgent. Exploring was her childhood; wonderful, free, roaming the riverbanks, searching for blackberries, tree climbing, and interacting with other children. Getting fiercely sunburnt or achingly cold depending on the season, but always happy and much loved, growing, and preparing for adulthood.

The only smudge on this utopian existence was the severe illness of her father, Jack James. He was a member of the Tenth Light Horse and fought in Egypt in World War 1. Although he was a solidly-built man, he had suffered a heart attack at the age of 45, and Gina remembered visiting him in the hospital. The long, narrow passages, nurses never walking but swishing hurriedly past in their white shoes and uniforms. Her father was lying heavily in the hospital bed – so ill he could hardly speak. Throughout it all, her mother had maintained an air of optimism, with no hint of fear or self-pity. So, it was only natural for them to expect that he should come home from the hospital to be a part of the family once more. But he was weak and unable to walk.

After dinner one evening – as was their custom – they gathered together, listening to the wireless. Gina sat by the fire with her parents and her brother, Jim. Mother was sewing, Jim was reading, and she was drawing. Her father was sitting in his comfortable cane chair. Suddenly there was a muffled moan, and her father slipped to the floor. Her mother fell to her knees and held her husband tightly. The thrombosis had struck, and her father died in the arms of his beloved wife. The hospital was unable to do any more and had sent him home to wait for just such an outcome.

Throughout the long night, neighbours, comforting relatives, and doctors created deep shadows, moving to and fro. There were no conversations, no sobbing, just movement, and silence. The undertaker must have been among the visitors that fateful night because, in the morning, a casket lay in the main bedroom. No one suggested she look upon her father, but she presumed she could if she wanted to. The solemnity of the occasion overwhelmed her, and she stood at the door, unable to move further and gazed in helpless sadness at the box.

The coffin disappeared. Gina did not attend the funeral. Nor did her mother or any of her aunties. It was certainly not a reflection of any lack of love, purely the custom in their family and their circle of friends. It was appropriate that only the men attend funerals. It was no place for women and children.

Life resumed, but to a slightly different pattern. Gina's mother was able to obtain clerical work – no mean feat considering that it was 1944 and the Second World War had not yet ended. With her mother being such a strong woman, there were no undue tears, anxiety, or drama. Life was lived a lot more among her aunties, which was pleasant enough, although she had noticed that the double bed in her parents' room had been replaced by a single bed – a single sadness, unable to be shared anymore.

Life bowled on, and their family built a life on a foundation of complete trust. School was over, and Gina had the office job her mother had so keenly advocated. Eventually, it was marrying time, and – like magic – *there he was!* Ralph Morgan: tall, dark, and handsome.

Ralph had been born a country boy, but the family had moved to the city for Ralph and his younger brother to receive a better education. Ralph was a brilliant man, and after studying at the university, he became an analytical chemist. Ralph was gentle of heart and kind in nature. Introductions had taken place between them, and friendship and romance blossomed, followed by marriage. There were no financial difficulties; they built their dream house and lived attuned to each other in harmony. How does one explain happiness? Ralph and Gina loved each other dearly and were kind, respectful, and considerate because they could not bear to hurt each other.

Gina remembered when she first fell pregnant. It had taken such a long time. Sickness plagued her, not just in the morning, but all day and night for the entire nine months of her pregnancy. It was a relief when Graham was born. A blue-eyed, blonde-haired, healthy little boy.

Her mother came to live with them, and life was good, but for the fierce longing to have another child. The next four years were miscarriage after miscarriage, and Gina's desire for another baby had turned into an ugly obsession that encroached upon all her waking moments. She desperately wanted a little girl, and every night when her head touched her pillow, she silently cried out to God in turmoil for Him to answer her prayer. Many a sleepless night was spent in anguish; tossing and turning, begging for her desperate plea to be heard and somehow become a reality. The ladies' group at church were studying the story of Hannah in the Bible. Her own emotions took her to the same place of Hannah's anguish.

Hannah was barren and desperately wanted a child, so she cried out to God for a baby boy. In her anguish to have a baby, she went to the temple every day and petitioned her deep longings. Hannah begged God to have mercy on her, and she made a vow to Him. Her promise and prayer were: *Oh God Almighty, if you will only see my misery and remember me by giving me a son, then I will give my son to serve you, God, for all the days of his life.*

Hannah's pain was so deep that her mouth moved, but no words came out. Eli, the priest, noticed her strange behaviour and thought she was drunk. He rebuked her. When he found out what her sincere request to God was, it moved him. On God's behalf, Eli blessed her, saying: "Go in peace, and may the God of Israel grant you what you have asked of Him." With time, Hannah gave birth to a son. She called him Samuel. Hannah was so thrilled that she made good on her promise and took Samuel to the temple to serve the Lord.

Gina identified deeply with Hannah's pain and decided in her heart that if God heard Hannah's cry, maybe God would listen to her cry too. Every night Gina prayed, "Lord, if you give me a child – and I want a little girl, but irrespective of the gender, I will dedicate this child to service unto you too," and every day she lived in hope.

After long talks, and heartbreaking debates about options, she and Ralph had decided on a way forward. As suggested by Dr Bray, they would now venture on the only path available to them: adoption.

"Gina Morgan," a voice echoed from reception. "The Doctor will see you now."

Gina liked Dr Bray. He had a warm presence, and Gina spoke comfortably. "Dr Bray, Ralph and I have talked about your suggestion. We are ready now. We want to adopt."

A look of delight appeared on his face as he looked over his little, round, silver-rimmed glasses and started shuffling through forms.

"Well, Gina, that's wonderful! It just so happens that at this very moment, I have a young lady in my care who wishes to put her baby up for adoption. She is a nice girl, from a reputable family, but unfortunately, someone has taken advantage of her. The baby is due to be born in the next few months, and it is at my discretion to recommend a placement, and I see no reason why you and Ralph should not have this child. Of course, we don't know what sex it will be – and I know you have your heart set on a little girl – but if you wish to have this baby when it is born, then it will be yours."

Gina could hardly believe what was happening. She felt lightheaded as if she was in a dream, and the words poured out of her effortlessly. "Yes, Dr Bray. Thank you so much! Of course, Ralph and I will have this child."

Dr Bray paused for a moment as he seemed to remember something. "Another lady has also seen me to adopt the next child." Pausing for another short moment, he spoke again, "But she *has* already adopted four." He opened a file and pulled out a completed application form. "It seems a bit unfair…"

Dr Bray appeared to be talking to himself as much as he was talking to her. He tapped his nose, winked, and put a new, blank *Request for Adoption* form on top of the completed one.

"Well, we won't say anything about that, will we?"

Gina stared at him in bewilderment and shook her head. In her eyes, Dr Bray had a sovereign authority similar to God, as he held the destiny of people in his hands. This morning had just proved it. Dr Bray had the power to place a life where-ever he chose.

He handed Gina the new form to fill in and gave her a nod and a smile.

Her hand floated across the pages, writing quickly. When she came to the end of the form to sign her name, overwhelming emotions rose, and she had to fight back a flood of tears.

Dr Bray, finalising the procedure said, "As I mentioned, the woman's baby is due in the next few months, which will take you up to the end of June. All you need now is to engage a lawyer to execute the legalities, and when the child is born, you will have your baby."

"Thank you, Dr Bray," Gina said with a heart full of gratitude. She was instantly filled with overwhelming joy. Her brother Jim had studied law and worked for a reputable firm, so she could use their services to process the adoption. It all seemed too easy.

Gina couldn't wait to get home and tell Ralph the fantastic news. As she drove home, she took a deep breath and let out a massive sigh of relief. She was deeply touched, and all the way home, she thanked God for answering her prayers.

"God, I know this baby is special and that you have given this child to me to look after. You have chosen me, and I am blessed. I will be forever grateful to you. I ask you to protect and keep this little child safe – all its life."

Gina did have a secret, hidden fear that the birth mother would have a change of heart and try to claim the baby back. There were horrible stories of this happening, and it was quite common. But she had to put that at the back of her mind. Right now, she had only the excitement, relief, and pleasure of one thing swirling around inside her, "I'm going to have a baby!"

When Gina arrived home, she cooked a fancy dinner for her and Ralph to celebrate the exciting news. Her mother bathed and fed Graham earlier so they could spend the intimate night alone.

Ralph walked through the door as usual and sensed the excitement radiating from his wife.

"My darling, what's the special occasion?"

Gina blew out the match she was holding and turned from the candle on the table.

"Ralph, I went and saw Dr Bray today."

"And?" he asked, eyes wide with anticipation.

"And… a child is available for adoption, and it is going to be ours!" she exclaimed.

Ralph took her in his arms and swung her around. "This is incredible news!"

He set her back on her feet and wrapped her in a hug.

"I'm so happy, Ralph," Gina said. "Are you?"

Ralph smiled widely. "It's wonderful! Yes, I'm happy, and I'm happy for you, my darling!" Ralph knew about Gina's tears and secret anguish.

They sat together, united in awe and wonder, and started planning for when their new baby would be part of their family.

In the weeks that followed, there were many unannounced visits and interviews by a social worker who came to check on their home life. It was such an invasion, and Gina quickly became fed up with the woman's lack of empathy and spying eyes.

More than once, the social worker made a stupid comment, which Gina suspected she said to every woman she visited.

"You know what will happen, don't you?" the woman said, "You'll adopt this baby, and then you'll probably fall pregnant. That's Murphy's law, isn't it."

Gina thought through her fake smile. *You are nothing but a stupid woman!* She always had to pretend she liked her. There was no way she would do anything to jeopardise their application.

Finally, their adoption was approved. Ralph and Gina passed the requirements – love, stability, and financial security. All they could do now was wait for the day their baby would enter the world and become part of their family.

This baby was about to be woven into Gina's tapestry of life, totally unaware of the threads of grief and sadness, excitement, and joy that were being unravelled and rewoven. Some ends were being cut off and finished, to introduce new threads. It was going to be an exciting and beautiful masterpiece, after all.

On the evening of the 29th of June 1962, the telephone rang in the Morgan household with an anticipated thrill. Gina reached out to pick it up – her hand was shaking.

Dr Bray's voice was full of celebration as he announced, "Congratulations, Gina and Ralph! You have a little *girl!*"

Gina burst into tears. "Thank you, Dr Bray. Thank you for everything you have done for us!" He had been pivotal in orchestrating this miracle.

Dr Bray made a profound statement, "*Gina, she was born to be yours!*" And Gina knew, with every fibre of her being, this was *a perfect destiny – for such a time as this.*

There were no more tears on Gina's pillow. As she lay down in bed that night, she thanked God with all her heart once again and made good on her promise. Gina prayed, "God, I dedicate this little girl *for service unto you* all the days of her life."

Ralph and Gina were instructed by Dr Bray to wait five days before they could attend the hospital. Firstly, to make sure that the baby had passed all her health checks and secondly to allow time for the birth mother to be released.

It was not uncommon for birth mothers who had offered their babies up for adoption to change their minds. With feelings of sincere regret, they would grab their baby and abandon the hospital. Also, there was a chance the birth mother would cross paths with the adopted parents, or even worse – see them holding her baby in their arms. Either would be a total disaster, leaving the hospital staff to deal with an emotional crisis.

Over the next five days, Gina lived in a dream. Arrangements were quickly made for them to bring their baby home, though, for Gina, the days crawled past excruciatingly slowly.

Finally, when the appointed morning came, Gina couldn't jump out of bed fast enough.

"Today's the day!" she exclaimed joyously to Ralph and began to race around in an excited daze.

"Yes, my darling," Ralph replied with a chuckle, "everything is more than ready for us to bring our little girl home. You have done wonders in preparing her room!"

"Oh, Ralph, I just want it all to be perfect!" Gina said, laying her best clothes on the bed.

"Just breathe my darling," Ralph reassured his wife, "just breathe, she will be in your arms very soon."

Ralph and Gina arrived at the hospital, and a young nurse ushered them into a very well-organised nursery where rows of cribs filled the room. Boys wrapped in blue blankets and girls in pink. She asked them to wait for Nurse Jacobs, so Ralph and Gina stood patiently. There was only one thing on Gina's mind – *which baby is mine?* Standing, waiting was torture.

Nurse Jacobs was finalising the baby's two birth certificates. On the first certificate, the baby had been named Mavis Patterson. Laurie used her mother's name to register the baby, and this was purely for legalities. As this was an adoption transfer, the second birth certificate counteracted the first one. By law, this second certificate was now the original birth certificate, and the baby's birth name would be whatever the adoptive parents chose.

The baby had been nameless for five days, and it bothered Nurse Jacobs. Taking the baby away from her mother was sad enough, but for her to see the baby with no identity, day after day, seemed to prolong the abandonment somehow. She was keen to write a name on the blank, white tag on the crib, and thankfully today, she would be able to do so.

The young nurse approached Ralph and Gina, "Nurse Jacobs is here now," she told them.

Gina gripped Ralph's hand. She felt herself starting to tremble.

Nurse Jacobs greeted them in a polite, professional manner, and Gina – her stomach turning in nervous excitement – promptly blurted out, "Which baby is mine?"

Nurse Jacobs gestured to a tiny baby wrapped in pink at the end of the row. "This one."

Still holding Ralph's hand, they walked over and peered into the cot. Tears welled up in Gina's eyes, and she spoke softly, "Ralph, look – our baby." Ralph acknowledged her delight with a gentle nod.

"Have you a name for her?" Nurse Jacobs asked, straight away. Aside from having a job to do, this tiny infant had touched her heart – she had been the only baby in the nursery without a name.

Gina took a breath to compose herself, looked up at Nurse Jacobs, and answered proudly, "She's Emma. Our little Emma Morgan."

Immediately Nurse Jacobs pulled a pen from her pocket and neatly wrote EMMA MORGAN on the crisp white card. Now this baby had an identity. Nurse Jacobs reached into the cot, took the baby carefully in her arms, looked at Gina, and said, "Here is your daughter, Emma."

She handed Gina the warm pink bundle. A wave of love and emotion flowed between Gina and her tiny new baby. She didn't ever want to let her go. Reluctantly, she passed Emma to Ralph, and then politely snatched her back as soon as she could. The desire to love and protect this child was so strong, the bond she could feel between them already was overwhelming.

The baby looked up at Gina's face. "Emma, do you like that name?" Gina asked softly. She marvelled at the baby's rosebud lips and her tiny, bright pink face. Her mop of brown hair was as soft as duckling's feathers. "What a miracle you are!" Gina stated proudly. Emma's little brown eyes looked directly into hers. It was as though a delicate halo of love had settled upon them both; a feeling of togetherness that was indescribable and unexplainable, but Gina felt it, and she knew Emma sensed it too. In that moment, they were indeed mother and child.

A nurse walked over to them and politely interrupted. She presented Gina with a handmade baby blanket and said, "This is for you and your baby. A lady makes these as a kind gesture for all the adopted babies who come through this hospital. There is a quote attached if you want to read it."

Gina took the blanket and thanked her. "It's lovely."

Her eyes glanced down at the card. It read: '*Not flesh of my flesh nor bone of my bone – but still miraculously my own. Never forget for a single minute, you didn't grow under my heart but in it.*' ~ *Fleur Conkling Heyliger.*

Reading the poem was too much for Gina, and now, overcome with emotion, she just wanted to get Emma home.

As Ralph and Gina left the nursery, another nurse mentioned that she had seen the birth mother, describing her as a tall woman with dark hair and eyes. Gina gracefully received the information, thinking it would be useful to be able to tell Emma about her birth mother in the years to come. But that will be much later, she thought, as a wave of fierce protectiveness rose inside her.

Gina looked down at her tiny, beautiful baby; her eyes now closed as she slept. She could hardly believe this baby was hers, but she was. Oh, how Gina loved her little girl. She whispered sweet affections over Emma's face as she carried her in her arms down the corridor and out of the hospital. "You were born to be mine, Emma. Do you know that?" It was a love story of its own. Gina knew deep in her heart God had blessed her. A warm, soft, tender essence settled upon them like a gift sent from heaven. Nothing or no one could ever break this incredible strand now weaving them together.

Emma opened her eyes as if to respond to the love cascading over her little being.

"Hello, Emma," Gina whispered, "I have so much to tell you, and your life with us has only just begun. But for now, I want you to know one thing. You are my baby, and I love you very much. I will look after you every day of your life, and you will get to know me. I will always love you. I am your mother, and you will always be my child."

CHAPTER 3

Childhood Days

"**G**randma, Grandma – help me!" I screamed a high-pitched squeal. Sheer terror pulsed through my body, and I was in full flight mode. Grandma was the only safe place in my home. "GRANDMA WHERE ARE YOU?!" I shouted.

My mind raced in turmoil. *Where can I hide? Where is she?*

Then I saw her, and I ran headfirst into her apron. It always surprised me that whenever I needed Grandma, she suddenly appeared out of nowhere.

"I'm here, Pet! What on earth is wrong?" Grandma wrapped her arms around me.

"Graham is after me again! He said he's going to punch me in the head until I'm dead!"

Grandma's words were soothing. "No, Pet, just stay with me, and you'll be all right."

"It's not just me, Grandma! It's my family! He's a horrible brother!" I was sobbing now.

"Which family this time? Your snails?" Grandma asked.

"Yes, all of them. I couldn't make Graham stop. Grandma, he's already done it!"

"Done what Pet. Tell me." Grandma held me tightly.

"He's cut the eyes off my snails again with the kitchen scissors! Every one of them screamed in pain, and now they can't see! And Graham just laughed!"

Grandma squeezed tighter, "Come now, Pet." Her voice was as soothing as a healing balm. "Let's sit down together, and you can tell me *all* about it!"

She held me close to her warm body. For now, I was safe. But there would always be a next time.

Graham didn't like me, but I never knew why. He found ways to bully and torment me – *every day*. Graham abused me physically, emotionally, and mentally. Cunningly, he lured me into his traps by saying he wanted to be my friend. Of course, in my little sister's childlike trust, I believed him.

I'm not sure what age I was when Graham's abuse started. My memories go as far back to when I was three, and Graham was seven, but it could have been earlier. I was always on the lookout to avoid *the enemy* who was out to get me. The house I lived in was my warzone. Family outings and holidays were my nightmares. Graham was smart, and his forms of torture were calculating and sly.

Graham invented an ingenious way to electrocute me on his car racing set, promising me it was safe, but I was never safe, and the shock waves were excruciating as they pulsed through my body. Then snidely, he would laugh and poke fun at my injuries for the rest of the day.

Mother was forever bandaging my wounds. Graham loosened the wheels on my trike once and then asked me for a race down the hill. Of course, it ended in disaster. Another time Graham spilt boiling water on me at bath time. He delighted in hurting me anyway he could and regularly set booby traps to scare me. Whenever Graham had the chance, he would hit me, pinch me or bang my head on the ground. Graham repeatedly punched me in the chest and jeered that my breasts would never grow and I was terrified they never would.

Even while I was cleaning my teeth or eating my breakfast, I always had to be on the lookout. Everyday Graham had some new and horrific torture he had devised for me, as I wouldn't fall for the same trick more than a few times.

He never called me by my name. When no one else was around, it was 'Pigatha.' A dirty, ugly pig! Graham managed to find a way to destroy everything dear to me, and then laugh and sneer in satisfaction.

This morning's premeditated attack was maiming my family of snails. I made friends with the creatures in the garden: snails, ants, and caterpillars. I gave them names and made them houses. I fed them and cared for them. Graham either stood on them with his big school boots – crushing them in one blow – or drowned them in the birdbath. I was forever grieving the loss of them. I know they were only insects, but to me, they were my family. All I wanted was a big brother to look after me and play with me, but we were like chalk and cheese.

I tried to tell Mother of Graham's abuse. I showed Mother my bruises from his schemes, but she would say calmly, "All big brothers tease their little sisters – just ignore him." I did try, but it was impossible.

Raised with a British mindset, we showed a stiff upper lip at all times. Show no emotion in the face of adversity, and eventually, the bad times will pass. Unfortunately, these bad times with Graham did not.

Grandma had lived with us ever since I was born. Just as well, because she was my refuge. Florence James was my mother's mother. She carried herself with quiet confidence. Her blue eyes sparkled with love and openness that made you feel like you were the most significant person in the whole world. She was always laughing and singing all the old-time songs, and occasionally tried her best with the modern ones, but forever got the words wrong.

Famous for her delicious Dutch cake – a spicy cinnamon mixture with a layer of jam and pastry on the bottom and topped with pink icing – Grandma cooked with love, and you could taste it! She never remarried after her husband died, her reason being, she loved him so much that no one would ever replace him. Apart from Mother, she was the kindest, most loving person I had ever known. We had our little secrets too.

One time I had been playing with Mother's makeup – as little girls do. The lid on the powder compact was stuck tight, and I failed to foresee that one swift pull would result in the apricot-coloured dust floating down all over Mother's white satin bedspread. On tiptoes and with whispers, Grandma and I cleaned it up immediately – saving me from a telling off.

I snuggled up to Grandma in her warm single bed and ate nougat. We used to play a game: whoever ate theirs the *slowest* got another one for later. Of course, I always watched intently, always a bite behind.

On occasion, she would let me try on her wedding ring. "It will be yours one day," Grandma would say, her voice filled with pride, and I couldn't wait for that day to come. To find a man who would love, protect, and keep me safe. I craved to be loved and protected.

My earliest childhood memory was on Christmas day. I would have been around one and a half years old and remember it like yesterday. My mind is like a movie camera. I remember events in my life as if I am watching a film. They call it a photographic memory, and I can't help thinking this ability was given to me to write the pages for this book.

I was standing in my safe cot when Dad came into my room with a bag of lolly coins. The gold foil sparkled as he unwrapped and revealed the sweet sticky disk. We each ate one, the chocolate oozing through my fingers. I remember bouncing up and down on my little legs, as I giggled with this man – who I adored.

Mother and I had a closeness far beyond the universal kinship for parent and child. I can't even write the words to describe our relationship. If I use the tapestry analogy, it would be something like this; the beautiful threads of Mother's unconditional love wove deep into the design of my fabric, tenderly embroidering a rare and precious bond to be cherished between us forever.

She loved me calling her Mother. I know it's old fashioned, but there was an absolute privilege in the tone and essence of her title. One she was proud to carry – *because of me.*

When I was a little girl, my beautiful dad would take me to the local football games on a Saturday afternoon to watch his footy team. Sitting with him on the benches and shouting out to the players was one of my favourite things to do with him, but we had other unique interactions.

After helping him in the garden, and having to wash our hands before lunch, my dad would get the sweet, scented soap and lather it up in his hands. After it frothed up into bubbles, it was my cue to place my little hands inside his. We would swirl them around together. His hands were soft and warm, and so large compared to mine. I felt loved and safe every time we did this.

Dad called me *Petal*. He had a natural love for the garden, and his favourite flower was the rose. I was his little rosebud and most precious blossom of all. My dad made me feel special.

Even though I had a brother, I grew up like an only child. When Graham went to play at his friend's houses, I was a happy little girl. It gave me a small window of time where I knew I could relax and be free in my own home without having to always look over my shoulder.

I also enjoyed going to Sunday School at the Uniting Church. My mother sang in the choir and was involved in the lady's meetings. I loved getting dressed up in my party dress and shiny red shoes every Sunday. The teachers were warm and loving and complimented me on just about everything I said and did. I remember being very proud of a colouring-in I had done in one of the lessons. It was of Jesus. He was the good shepherd and held a staff in His hand as He looked after the little lambs that were gathered all around Him. I remember thinking: *those lambs are very lucky. Jesus loves them and is looking after them. I like Jesus!*

Mother and Dad had me baptised, in their church, when I was one year old. They saw it as their Christian duty to dedicate my life officially to the Lord so that He would be the good shepherd of my life too. Mother always told me there was a loving God in heaven, ready to hear my prayers. A distant connection was the extent of my relationship with God when I was a child, and although it was quite simple, it was a security.

One of my favourite things to do was to pretend I was Cinderella going to the ball. Mother had read the story to me enough times that I knew it off by heart. I would go downstairs into the laundry room and find the old mop. When I turned it the wrong way up, it made a very respectable Prince Charming, who was only a little bit taller than me. I would take a curtsy, and he would bow, and then he would embrace me in his arms, and we would waltz around the laundry floor in circles, spinning and laughing out of true love and delight. It was my deep longing. To be loved and cherished – just for being me.

Every year our school put on a gala event. I was in grade two, and our class recited a poem about Jim, who went to the zoo and got eaten by a lion. My memory skills were sharp, so I learned this very quickly.

Our second performance was a dance to the Cinderella story. Each girl was a Cinderella, and each boy her dashing prince. At rehearsals, we skipped and spun to the music. It was so much fun. My prince had sweaty hands, but I didn't care.

Our teacher drew up patterns, and every mother made their daughter an apron out of crepe paper. A brilliant design as they were reversible. In the dance routine, when we swept the floors as poor Cinderella, the apron was plain and dull, but as soon as it was time to go to the ball, we quickly turned it around, and the apron displayed elaborate frills and glittering jewels.

After weeks of rehearsals, the gala-night arrived, and all the students from every year gathered in the great assembly hall. Most students had brought their parents. It was a full house, and class by class, we watched and clapped, thoroughly entertained.

Soon it was our turn – everyone *ooooh-ed* and *ahhh-ed* in all the right places when the lion devoured poor Jim. Now for Cinderella! Scene one – the girls took the stage wearing the drab aprons, spinning around in circles to the music while sweeping with a broom. I felt like I was one of the best because I danced at home in the laundry. On cue – when the music stopped – the girls ran to the side, and with a quick turn-around of our aprons, we entered back onto the stage. Our jewelled sparkles made a great impression as loud gasps resounded from the audience.

The boys walked swiftly out onto the stage, handsomely dressed in pants, shirts, and sparkly bow ties to match his Cinderella's beautiful apron. Everyone was ready and in position for the grand display of joyful spins to commence – everyone except me. My partner had not turned up. I had no prince. Panic rose inside me, and I ran off the stage to tell the teacher I had no partner. She panicked as well and became extremely angry. She pushed me back onto the stage, saying, "Dance by yourself!"

The lights came on, the music started, and out of the corner of my eye, I saw the boys whizzing the girls around performing our rehearsed routine. I had no choice but to join in with them, holding my arms up in the air, pretending I had someone. Except I was by myself. Utterly embarrassed and humiliated by the rejection, I felt alone and unwanted. I heard people laughing, and I was sure they were laughing at me. I did my best to hold back my tears so that I wouldn't cry on stage, and the music seemed to play forever. Finally, *finally*, there was a great round of applause. The girls curtsied, and the boys bowed, and we walked promptly off the stage.

When I got home, of course, Graham teased me. He told me that my prince hadn't turned up because I was so ugly. I never found out the reason why my partner didn't come, but as a little girl, I believed what Graham said. I *must* be ugly!

With this repeated belief, a great fear took hold of me and a sinister voice whispered, '*You will never find true love, and your prince will never turn up to love, hold and protect you.*' This voice became a familiar sound as it seeped into my mind and reinforced my doubts and fears every day.

My birthday parties were always one of my favourite days of the year, and Mother and Grandma planned them weeks in advance. We played games such as apple on a string, passing the parcel, treasure hunt, fancy dress-up race, memory tray, and musical chairs before sitting down to jellied oranges, fairy bread, little red sausages and sauce, and – as always – a surprise birthday cake.

Our dog Patches had to be tied up outside, or she would eat the food right out of everyone's hands. It was always a successful day, but more than that, for me, it was a whole day off from Graham's abuse. He had no opportunity to taunt me, at least until they had all gone home.

Every night, at bedtime, after Mother prayed the Lord's prayer with me, Grandma came and tucked me in. Grandma would talk about the day and how precious I was. I wanted to know why both my little fingers were so crooked at the tips, but no one had an answer – other than I was special and unique – like a snowflake.

I always wondered why Graham was so mean to me, and I didn't feel special at all. I couldn't escape the feeling I didn't belong in this family or with anyone. I was a square peg in a round hole. My life had an empty feeling – of a limbo existence – which never left my thoughts or emotions. I had no deep sense of belonging anywhere. But my parents and Grandma loved me and told me often. And I loved them.

One place I did feel loved was when I played with my friend Rex. Rex – Judy's dog – was a handsome beagle. His coat was glossy, and his nature was typically loving. I was proud to say that of all the dogs I knew – even my dog, Patches – Rex was my favourite. We had an extraordinary bond. I loved going to Judy's house because I could spend time with my most faithful companion.

"Rex is out the back!" Judy told me when we arrived.

Judy knew that Rex loved me just as much as I loved him. I pushed open the flywire door and saw him lying down in the middle of the lawn. He had his back to me, so I thought that instead of calling him, I'd surprise him. Surprises with best friends are so much better! I tip-toed up behind him and flung both my arms around his neck. *The rest is black.*

They say your body copes with shock by going into a numbed state, and your mind blocks out trauma by turning the lights off in your brain. When I say black, I mean black. No memory. No feeling.

Nothing. I am telling you this from here as my mother has relayed it to me. I have no recollection of this ever happening.

Rex had been eating a bone. He must have dug up an old one because Judy hadn't given him one that day. I had given him a terrible fright by throwing my arms around him and reacting out of instinct; Rex just protected what was his. He defended his territory and snapped at my face.

His teeth bit right through my flesh from the top of my forehead to the bottom of my chin. His bite scraped deep into my cheeks, and his bottom teeth sunk and embedded into the roof of my mouth. Mother rushed me to the hospital. The doctor pushed my skin back into place and wrapped a long, white bandage around my head and face. The spectrum of my bruising was black, blue, yellow, orange, red, green, and purple – nearly all the colours of the rainbow.

The doctor stated my young skin should be repaired without too many scars. I healed without stitches, but where the skin was torn deeply around my mouth, scars were still visible. Graham now had new ammunition to tease me and told me my face was *even more ugly*. I was an impressionable five-year-old, and if my brother said I was ugly, then it must have been true.

The saddest of all – Rex was put to sleep. He had snapped at the neighbour's little girl the week before. She must have pulled his ears or something because he would never hurt anyone. My best friend – Rex – had died, and it was all my fault.

Despite this attack, my deep love for dogs remained, and I was never frightened of hugging any dog I met. I was thankful for the black.

I was more frightened of Graham than of dogs. Although I was afraid of many things, one fear loomed over me, night after night.

My wardrobe phobia!

Every night Grandma tucked me in, and before she left my bedroom, I insisted that she check the wardrobe door. The thought of the wardrobe door open – even a crack – sent me into an uncontrollable panic. Destructive dark thoughts gripped my mind, and I couldn't breathe. An evil presence swirled above me, taunting me, and I felt as though I was going to be swallowed down into a black abyss of torment forever, never to return. Without exaggeration – this was the intensity of fearing the wardrobe door might be open!

And it was a beautiful wardrobe – a white, Queen Anne style with an oval mirror and a fancy lock and key. Dad had gone to the hardware store and chosen plastic flower trimmings. He then spray-painted them gold and glued them all around the edge to form a pattern. It was feminine and a lovely piece of furniture. But to me, behind the door, concealed a black vortex of doom. No one, including me, knew how this phobia had come upon me. Mother and Grandma asked me many times if anything scary or hurtful had happened involving my wardrobe. Every time my answer was the same. No.

The wardrobe door phobia ruled my life. Every night, my bedtime routine went something like this:

In a panicked tone, I asked, "Grandma, is the wardrobe door shut tight?"

Grandma would walk over and show me the door was indeed fully closed. Her answer, "Yes, Pet, it's shut tight, now get some sleep."

"Are you sure?" Still fighting against the tsunami of fear drowning me.

"Yes, Pet, I'm certain!" Grandma reassured me by rechecking it.

"Thank you. Good night Grandma. I love you."

Grandma's voice always calmed me. "I love you too, Pet."

Knowing the door was shut caused my anxiety to subside and made my panic go away.

Grandma also had a quote she would recite with a chuckle in an attempt to alleviate my distress. "Don't let the bed bugs bite!" But nothing succeeded in taking away my ingrained fear.

Graham made sure he passed by my room each night to poke his head through my doorway, and in his scariest voice whispered: "Watch out Pigatha, the Larmings and the Plung-Gutchers are going to get you in the night and tear you to shreds!"

Graham's taunts raised a frantic call for Grandma or Mother to come and reassure me they were on the lookout for such creatures. I was terrified to fall asleep in case they came, and every night my dreams turned into nightmares. We never knew how the Larmings and the Plung-Gutchers came to be. I had made them up. Maybe I was *alarmed* these monsters Graham projected at me were going to *plunge and get me?* The Larmings and the Plung-Gutchers were Graham's allies, and he deployed his monster army against me very well.

One night, instead of a nightmare, I had a beautiful dream, unlike any I'd had before. I was six years old at the time. It took place at school. The home bell rang, and all the parents collected their children, but no one came for me. It grew dark, and I became scared. I noticed a red phone booth in the playground, and I walked over to it and stepped inside. The phone rang, so I picked it up.

"Hello!" There was no one there. Total darkness surrounded me, and I was alone and frightened. I saw someone walking towards me, and I felt instant peace. Who was this person? As He got closer, I saw that it was Jesus. He walked towards me with love and acceptance, and immediately in my heart, I knew that everything in my life was going to be all right. In the morning, when I awoke, I was still peaceful. Even at age six, I had a strong sense that if ever I was afraid, I would never have to face it alone. Jesus would always come for me.

In grade one, a particular instance at school affected me so dramatically; it changed the very existence of my life. We had to draw a picture of all the members of our family and colour them in. When my friend saw my drawing, she asked me a simple question, "Why does Graham have blonde hair and blue eyes, and your hair and eyes are brown?" Although this is quite common in families, I didn't have an answer for her.

Her question consumed me, and I thought about nothing else all day. Is this why I don't fit in anywhere? As soon as the last school bell rang, I ran all the way home thinking that Mother might know.

By the time I burst through the front door, that simple question now had become an obsession – an intense desire to know the answer. Mother was startled by my explosive countenance as I cried out, *"Mother! Why does Graham have blonde hair, and mine is brown?"*

Mother was still for a moment, before taking a deep breath, and then – quite composed – she looked straight at me and said calmly, "I knew this day would come. Yes, there is a reason."

I remember it as if it were yesterday. Mother sat me down on her knee and wrapped both arms around me and held me tightly. All I wanted to know was why Graham and I were so different. I sat in anticipation of her answer. She took another deep breath. I sat patiently and didn't move. And then, in a gentle, loving voice, she told me, "Emma, you had another mummy and daddy before dad and me. You came from another mummy's tummy. She loved you very much, but your other mummy and daddy couldn't look after you, and dad and I could. We wanted you so very much with all our hearts because you are just so special."

The only world I knew suddenly crashed violently around me. Instantly, I felt dizzy and sick. I sat in silence, stunned and numb. From here on, my memory plays in slow motion. Mother's words were comforting, although I had to focus hard on what she was saying. No matter how many times Mother emphasised the words *love, wanted, for my sake, special* – there was only one truth I absorbed which swirled around in my six-year-old brain. *I was so ugly and horrible that even my real mummy and daddy didn't want me!* I ran to my room, slammed the door, and sobbed. Without knowing it – massive rejection – in full force and completely uninvited – entered me.

Mother gave me more cuddles and affection, but no matter how many times she told me I was loved, I couldn't believe it. It was just too huge for my childlike mind to understand and process. The screams inside my head were piercing. *YOU WERE NOT WANTED!*

Everything Graham said about me was right! I was ugly, unwanted and unlovable, and these kind people only looked after me because they felt sorry for me. Why am I so ugly and such a nothing? I hated myself so much that at the age of six, I didn't want to live anymore.

These destructive feelings never went away. They only grew over the years. Graham's daily taunts increased too, and there was never any escape. My inner and outer worlds were always at war. Whenever Graham said, "You are so ugly, and no one will ever love you," I believed him to my core. I was not only tormented by him but also tormented by my thoughts, shouting at me with booming screams of self-hate, saturating my mind. These inner voices cemented this *as fact* into my brain. Layer upon layer of negative words and emotions, day in and day out, bound me to a place of darkness I couldn't escape.

Mother said she wished she had never told me I was adopted as I was never the same little girl again. The social worker had told my parents that six is the right age to say to a child they are adopted. Any younger and the child can't understand, any older, and it becomes too hard to comprehend as if their life has been a lie. In my opinion, I don't think any age is the right age to tell a child they are adopted. At any time of your life, it is an incredible shock.

My parents gave me double the love for my devastation; overseas holidays, fashionable clothes, jewellery, pets and they supported me in every activity I did. Their kindness was overwhelming. Nothing made up for my misery. Money and things couldn't replace how I felt about myself. My days became a roller-coaster of emotions, and I veered from extreme highs to the lowest of lows.

For me, being adopted was isolating. I felt like a lone undiscovered island in this world. There was only me who looked and acted like me. I couldn't place myself with another face or human being. Did I take after my mum or my dad? Did I have other brothers or sisters? I couldn't identify with anyone. Where did I belong? I didn't belong anywhere.

Mother noticed what a timid and nervous child I was becoming. A teacher highlighted in my grade one report, 'Emma worries over every little thing.' The teacher light-heartedly mentioned to my mother that if I kept going on like this – when I grew up, I would be a professional worrywart! My condition was nothing more than a topic of jest as they had no answers or understanding of my hidden mental state.

In today's society – with the growing knowledge and awareness of mental health issues – I would possibly be assessed and diagnosed with childhood trauma, depression, and anxiety and be given some support to cope. But back in the '60s, no one knew anything about such matters, and there was only one thing that soothed my pain.

"It's toddy time, Pet!" Grandma would call, holding out my delicate, butterfly-etched, crystal glass.

"Yummy, I'm here, Grandma!" I would reply, excited for our daily ritual.

Grandma had toddy time at four o'clock every afternoon. It wasn't just nougat I shared with her. Now, this delicious drink – McWilliams Sherry. It was socially acceptable in our well-to-do family for a child to have a little *drop of the doings* at dinner parties and special events. Mother never knew I had it with Grandma every day. Sipping this sweet syrup was another one of our secrets.

And I would also go and sneak it whenever I wanted it. I soon discovered, whenever I felt sad, I needed only a mouthful to make me feel warm and fuzzy and numb my pain, for a little while anyway. So, I guess you could say I started drinking alcohol every day from the age of six. It was my medicine and my escape from my mental anguish.

It was during the year of grade two at primary school. A visiting nurse came into our class to do a routine eyesight test. We stood in a line, and one by one, we walked up to a yellow mark and read – to the best of our ability – the eye chart, starting with E at the top and down to as far as we could go. When it was my turn, I stepped up to the mark and waited. After a nod from the nurse to proceed, I just stood there.

"Get on with it!" she said impatiently.

She was very frustrated at having to be there and had no tolerance for working with little children. Her annoyance with the chatter and giggles in the background was evident by the way she glared and hushed the row of tiny, excited, skinny-legged students. She seemed to want to get out of there as quickly as possible.

"Well, go on, don't just stand there. Read the chart!" the nurse snapped.

"I can't see it," I replied, thinking I was going to get into trouble.

"What do you mean you can't see it?" she snapped again.

Quietly I answered, "It's all blurry." All I could see was grey smudges in blobs.

"Well, take a step forward," she told me.

My legs were shaking with fear from her ferocious demeanour, but I obliged. Even more nervously, I said, "I still can't see."

I couldn't even pretend I did. The letters were just one big fuzzy mess.

"Oh, for goodness sake child, I haven't got time to waste on you! Take another step forward!" she said, her frustration escalating.

After five steps forward, I was only a metre away from the chart. I could see a large E, F, and P, but struggled with the letters after that and got most of them wrong.

"Good. Next!" the nurse called and waved me to go.

I thought it was strange; she made me move forward, but none of the other children did. But I was only seven, so I trusted and believed the taller and older people that surrounded me.

I had headaches nearly every day. Mother took me to the doctor, but he could see nothing physically wrong with me. I switched to soy milk as one of Mother's friends suggested that full cream milk might be the culprit. It was sour and tasted like crushed chalk and didn't relieve the pain in my head anyway. I lived on *Aspirin* every day, and where most little girls have a drawer full of hankies and plastic jewels, I had my pharmaceutical supply of pain relief.

Boxes of *Aspirin* were a part of my life.

I became a keen netball player. Dad fixed a goal ring up in the backyard, and I practiced every day. Weekly training kept me fit but walking home after practice in the winter months became a problem for me.

I only had to walk from the local oval to our house, but at dusk, the blurred trees swayed in the chilly wind. They took on shapes of people and convinced me strange and dangerous men were chasing me. No one ever grabbed me. There wasn't ever anyone there. I was as blind as a bat. People's faces were a blur – anything more than one metre away, I couldn't distinguish. I lived not in the sharpness of black and white and colour. I lived in the existence of *a blurred grey.*

In grade five, Mother received a phone call from the school. My teacher reported me for disrupting the class, talking, cheating, and being defiant towards her. Mother defended me to the hilt, with a face-off with the Principal. She knew this was totally out of my character and wouldn't believe anyone before getting to the truth of the matter and speaking to me about it first. When I got home from school, she posed the question to me directly.

"Emma, your Principal, phoned today and said you have been talking in class and copying the work of the person next to you, is this true?"

Under all circumstances, Mother told me to tell the truth, so I replied honestly, "Yes, I have to!"

Mother was confused. "Why do you have to?"

It was apparent to me. "Because I can't see the blackboard."

I had never been able to see the board any day at school for five years. Mother nearly fell off her chair. She couldn't believe what she was hearing. Instead of scolding me, which she had expected I may need, she grabbed me and hugged me. She cried tears of guilt and remorse for not realising herself that I couldn't see, and this was the cause for all my headaches. After a quick explanation to the Principal and a trip to the optometrist, Mother cried all the way home as I exclaimed with excitement how I could read the street signs and the number plates on the cars as if they had magically appeared for the first time to me in my world.

Graham named me blowfly-head, and at school, I got called four eyes. Whenever they could, my classmates made fun of me, holding their circled fingers up to their eyes. There were no anti-bullying campaigns in the '70s and teasing and punching were rife in schools. Reading, writing, arithmetic, and bullying were part of the curriculum. Only the strongest survived, and the top dogs led the pack with a fierce gang mentality. I was a target because I wore glasses and was timid. I was easy prey, ripe for the picking.

Wearing glasses added to my lack of confidence and automatically moulded my socially awkward body language, which stood out a mile. I hated myself so much because I believed, to my core, that I was ugly and unlovable. I truly wanted to die. Plagued with thoughts of suicide, I tried to overdose on *Aspirin* so I wouldn't hurt anymore. I only succeeded in making myself sick. I was nine years old.

Over the next few years, I was an emotional roller-coaster, mixed with happy family moments and Graham's daily psychological ridicule. His abuse continued until I reached about the age of 14. Graham got his car licence and wasn't home much. His social life was the beginning of my relief. But any respite for me now was too late. Permanent damage had already been done and established unhealthy cycles of self-hate and worthlessness in every part of me.

Alcohol was my only comfort, though it was a double-edged sword. The drinking fuelled my self-hate even more. Anxiety and depression trapped me in a dark cycle I couldn't break.

At 14, I was desperate for love and affection. Graham had told me every day how ugly I was. I just wanted to be beautiful. Maybe if I could find a man to love me as my Grandma did, then I wouldn't hurt anymore? Then I would be happy. That was it! I was determined to find a man who would love and protect me forever and relieve me from this painful state in which I lived.

CHAPTER 4

My Friend Jacky

Jacky and I clicked the first time we met at a combined family picnic. Our parents were friends through mutual acquaintances, and even though we lived in different suburbs, by a happy coincidence, we attended the same Ladies Private High School.

Jacky was 17 and I was 14. It felt *cool* to have an older friend. She had friends with cars and knew groups of boys. Life suddenly became exciting.

We had something else unusual in common – we were both adopted. Jacky also had an older brother, Dean, and – like Graham and I – they, too, were like chalk and cheese. Dean was the school jock; he was good at sports and incredibly good looking, and he knew it. His superior, up-himself nature led him to bully Jacky, and this extended to me when I slept over at their house. Jacky wasn't close to her adoptive parents like I was with mine. They were always finding fault with her, and they were constantly arguing. Her list of disappointments seemed never-ending.

Jacky's personality was extremely loud and bubbly, but the real force behind this was her low self-esteem and her self-hate. Prominent freckles covered her whole body, a perfect match for her bright red hair. She was very overweight and had braces on her teeth. Of course, she got teased a lot for all of these things.

Outwardly, Jacky appeared happy – and at school, she was the class clown – but because I knew her so well, she was an emotional time bomb, quietly ticking away, waiting to explode.

My parent's friendship circle organised a holiday to Rottnest Island. The teenage boys conspired together and stole Jacky's huge DD cup bra and hung it between two trees with a hand-made sign; HAMMOCK, FREE TO TRY. Of course, everyone knew it belonged to Jacky. She ripped it down and pretended not to care, but later that night, alone in the chalet, she ate a dozen doughnuts. Our parents suspected the quokkas had eaten them, but I knew it was Jacky. She was crying inside to be loved and accepted, not knowing who she was in this world either.

We bonded through what we didn't have, and while we shared the same rejection, I didn't know how to help Jacky. I didn't know how to help myself. Jacky soothed her inner pain with food, and I eased my emotional turmoil with alcohol. I would sneak my vice from my parent's liquor cabinet at any opportunity.

I had frequent outbursts of anger and always shouted at Mother at full force. Things like, "I wish you never adopted me!" and, "I hate you!" Of course, I didn't mean to hurt her, but for me, it was a release.

Mother always answered back, "Well, I'm glad I adopted you, and I love you." I hated myself even more for being so horrible to her.

I blamed my adoption for all my feelings of frustration and rejection.

Rejection is an evil beast. It eroded me away internally and forced me to believe I was insignificant. Nobody wanted to choose me. *Nobody will ever love me.*

Rejection then knocked on the door of depression, and together they ran rampant inside me. I lived in a state of constant emotional turmoil. Desperate to be accepted, I made myself vulnerable to draw in such a love from people. And when they did start to love me, I couldn't receive it. I believed I didn't deserve it.

I kept the people I wanted to love me at arms' length, in case they rejected me. I made sure I kept them shut out while I stayed safe behind my wall of protection.

No matter how hard I tried to find my joy in life, I was always unhappy. Unhappy because I was lonely. Miserable because I would never be good enough. Full of distress because I had made the walls of my own Fort Knox far too high for anyone to scale.

The only enemy was myself, and I secretly hated who I was. I put on my best smile for the world while I cried silently and continually on the inside. Torment was my secret daily life, and I suspected it was Jacky's too.

Jacky had another group of friends who invited us to an Easter Camp that year. The Uniting Church ran it, so it was going to be religious. We didn't care. Boys would be going, and that's all that mattered to us. Our teenage girl hormones were developing at a rapid pace, and male energy was fast becoming our only focus. Anywhere there would be boys, we would be there too. And since I was on my personal and desperate quest to find forever love, I was going to the Easter Camp with a hopeful expectation.

CHAPTER 5

Hello Supernatural

Jacky and I had been to a few of the Friday night youth gatherings, which had been fun, but this was going to be my first youth camp, and I didn't know what to expect. Frank, a young man who was a youth Pastor with the Uniting Church, ran the meetings. There was, on average, about 15 girls and guys who attended regularly.

Jacky and I were very excited to be having this weekend adventure together. This year the location was a campsite by the beach at Point Peron. Being the month of April, the weather was perfect. And yes, to my delight – *lots of boys were going!*

After meeting at the church, we climbed aboard a charter bus and set off for our adventure. I spied a cute boy sitting a few seats away from me. I casually asked around and found out his name was Ken. He had a solid build, blonde hair, and blue eyes. For me, it was love at first sight. I tried to get his attention, but he always looked past me. I said a little prayer – *please, God let me find love here at camp.*

Everyone was happy and friendly, and after an enjoyable road trip, Jacky and I settled into the girls' dorm. It was a large, cosy, timber chalet. There were four beds to a room, and we each had a little chest of drawers to hold all our belongings. My mattress and pillow were only just acceptable, considering this was camp comfort, and – most importantly – there were no wardrobes. I didn't need to worry. I always scanned new places to make sure I could cope with the surroundings. No wardrobes – now, I could relax.

After a typical camp-style dinner, we bunked down for the night in our dorm, with lights out at 10 o'clock. Jacky and I awoke in the morning to the sound of whispers from the other girls in our room.

Apparently, through the night, there had been a prowler peeping through the windows of our dorm. Some had suspected it was Eddie – an unfortunate-looking boy. His facial features were very pointy, which made him look extremely abnormal. His hair was long and matted, and he always wore the same dirty, tatty old t-shirt. In winter, he pulled on an old hand-knitted jumper which was just as soiled.

Eddie came to the youth group meetings, though most of us had never seen him, as he would only appear in the distance. His bike was his only companion. He wanted human connection, but he didn't know how to go about it. Eddie didn't speak. He only ever grunted. We understood he had a brain disorder, which caused him to flick his head from side to side. His eyes were black pinholes, and being around him or even looking at him, was scary.

Eddie didn't attend school. Instead, he spent his days riding around the streets. I think hanging around the fringes of the youth group was his way of being part of something. Eddie wasn't officially enrolled to come to camp, but without anyone knowing, he had secretly followed the bus on his bike.

A couple of the boys were very sure it was him slinking around looking in the windows of the girls' dorm and reported it to Frank. Although Eddie was known to be harmless, all the girls were frightened, in case he came back to spy through the window again. So, for the remainder of camp, it was organised two boys at a time would take turns to keep a look-out in rotation for the whole night. Of course, we girls thought this was very heroic.

It was now day two, and everyone was ready to get involved in the program. The first activity was to teach us appreciation.

We assembled in the main hall for lunch to find a row of tables joined together and set out like a wedding banquet. White cloths, silver cutlery, elaborate candlesticks, and pretty flowers all decorated the long table. It was fit for a king and queen. In front of this beautiful display, hessian sacks lay scattered on the hard floorboards.

One by one, names were drawn out of a box. The winners were all called forward and then led by the arm like royalty to sit at the table, while the remaining others – myself included – were ushered to squat on the floor on the harsh, prickly mats.

Quickly the kitchen staff rallied and set down fancy food before the chosen people who were to dine at the banquet. Dish after dish of prawns, chicken, beef, vegetables, and salads. Far too much for them to eat. Then, delicious desserts. Cheesecake, cream puffs, ice cream, and chocolate mousse were all presented politely to them.

We squatters on the floor were simply onlookers. It stirred our hunger even more. Then after a long wait, our lunch finally came. A small, raw cabbage leaf for our bowl containing half a cup of cooked white rice. What? We couldn't believe the unfairness. With unwashed hands, we scooped up the sticky, bland, tasteless, unsatisfying substance into our mouths. When we had finished, we were free to go. The people on the banqueting table couldn't eat all their food, so the excess was thrown in the bin. Those of us who were on the floor would have gladly taken the scraps. It was a lesson in gratitude and to help broaden our minds to the reality of some people's lives in the world. It impacted me greatly, and it is an experience I have never forgotten.

Straight afterwards, it was free time. I'm sure this was done on purpose so we could reflect. I wondered what Ken was doing. I was starving and didn't know what to do with myself. I couldn't find Jacky. She had gone off for the group walk, so I decided to hang around the girl's dorm with Leanne, a new friend I had made. She was so lovely and gave me some lollies she had in her backpack. I was hungry and grateful, and after our lesson of rice and cabbage, even more so.

We sat on the grass under the shade of a massive peppermint tree outside the dorm.

The sunshine was gentle and warm. I loved perfect autumn days, and this was one of them.

Leanne opened her heart and shared how something was always missing in her life. She explained that at the youth group, she learned about God's love and gave her heart to Jesus. It was only after doing this her life started making sense. Jesus made her feel complete, and she had true inner fulfilment.

"Do you know much about God?" Leanne asked.

"My mother has told me that God is love, and He hears my prayers," I replied.

Leanne had her Bible with her and asked me, "Can I read you some scriptures?" I nodded, thinking our time together was lovely. Leanne read, "John 3 verse 16, 'For God so loved the world that He gave His one and only son, that whoever believes in Him shall not perish but have eternal life.'"

I sat and listened to the sound of her soft voice. It was very soothing. Leanne turned to another scripture. "Romans 10 verse 9, 'that if you confess with your mouth, Jesus is Lord, and believe in your heart that God raised Him from the dead, you will be saved'. Do you know Emma, when someone prayed with me years ago, Jesus became my best friend? He fills me daily with His love, and I am never alone."

ALONE! That last word struck me deep down inside. My whole life, I always felt alone. Leanne had a presence that put me at ease. I knew I could trust her even though she was somewhat a stranger. I told her about my dream with Jesus and the phone booth when I was six. I shared, "Leanne, *I always feel alone.*"

She paused and asked, "Would you like me to pray for you?"

No one had ever asked me if they could pray for me before. It was lovely.

"Yes, I'd like that!" I replied.

Leanne took both my hands in hers, and I closed my eyes. Her prayer was gentle; her words soothing. She paused again and then asked me if I wanted to ask Jesus into my heart.

Without knowing very much about God, it just felt right.

I answered, "Yes, Leanne, I will."

Her grip on my hands became firmer as she straightened up. "Emma, just say this from your heart."

Leanne spoke, and I repeated after her, line by line, "Father God, thank you for sending Jesus your son to die for me. I believe Jesus, you are the Son of God, and You died and rose again to take away my sins. Forgive me for all my sins. Thank you for washing away my sins as I repent from them now. Fill me with your Holy Spirit and let your peace always lead me into the truth of God's love for me. Amen."

Leanne hugged me and said, "Congratulations, Emma, you are now officially a Christian. Woohoo!"

I felt a substantial peace settle around me and then a warm, tangible essence flooded right through to the core of my being. *Something had just happened on the inside of me.* I had gone to Sunday school and learned about Jesus, but why hadn't I known about this before? I never knew it was possible to ask Jesus into my heart, have my sins forgiven, and be filled with a deep, *deep* peace. Leanne was right! Receiving God's love was the most *INCREDIBLE* experience!

I spent the rest of the afternoon sitting by myself under the shade of that enormous peppermint tree feeling calm, and for the first time in my life, totally content and fulfilled.

I was starving hungry by dinner time, and after another hearty camp meal – one I was even more grateful for – I decided to go to bed a bit earlier than everyone else. It had been quite an emotional day sharing with Leanne, and I was tired. As I climbed into my sleeping bag, I couldn't stop thinking about how beautiful and peaceful I felt after asking Jesus to come into my heart. I rolled over, trying to get comfortable on the semi-hard mattress. Instantly, I was startled! A man was sitting at the end of my bed. I panicked and immediately thought – *oh my goodness, it's Eddie, the prowler!* He was sitting side on to me and was looking down at the floor.

The man – sensing my fright – looked up at me, and I heard His soft words, "*It's all right, it's me, Jesus.*"

A tangible wave of peace flowed over me. The same peace I had felt earlier that day. I had no explanation as to how I was seeing Him, but very clearly, *I was seeing Jesus.* He wore a grey, long-sleeved shirt, and grey pants, and was also barefoot. He had shoulder-length brown hair and a beard. If humbleness could be a garment, He would be wearing that as well. His demeanour was pure humility.

We had a brief conversation. The only way I can describe it is that it was from – Spirit to spirit. We spoke no actual words.

Silently from my heart, I said, "*Thank you for what happened today, Jesus. It was amazing! This peace, I feel – that you give to me! It's incredible!*"

Jesus looked at me and smiled. His face was kind, soft, and loving. I could tell by His radiant countenance; He was happy as well.

I was so full of deep joy and peace – I could burst. I felt content and safe. Then Jesus looked down at His feet, deep in thought. He appeared worried. It was as though He knew something unfortunate that I didn't, but He couldn't tell me.

Jesus looked up, turning His face towards me again, and with such tenderness, I heard, "*I will never leave you; I will never forsake you.*"

His words seared my heart – like a promise – He would never break. His love was so strong it frightened me, and yet, I felt overwhelmingly safe at the same time. I nodded my head towards Him, and if even at all possible, I entered an even more profound peace.

As I closed my eyes, my spirit replied, "*Thank you, Jesus.*"

Overcome with what had just happened, I thought to myself – Leanne forgot to tell me Jesus would appear the day I gave my heart to Him. I assumed this was a normal part of the procedure. You give your heart to Jesus – and then He comes and tells you – He will never leave you or forsake you. I had no idea at the time – at the age of 14 – God was setting the stage for a future scene to unfold in the later years of my life. Another strong wave of peace flowed over me, and I drifted off to sleep, thinking this had all been very lovely.

There were tears and hugs at the end of camp. It had been the best thing I had ever done in my life. It didn't bother me; Ken hadn't noticed me. God answered my prayers, and *I had* found the love of a man. A man named Jesus. His passion for me was pure, authentic, and forever. I never saw Jesus again the way I saw Him that night, but I could feel Him close to me, and I knew God was only a prayer away. I didn't feel alone anymore. Jesus was with me all the time. His Spirit gave me a glowing inner strength, and for the very first time in my entire life, I felt I could accept myself.

As I waved my goodbyes, I promised Leanne I would join the youth group. I shared with Jacky I had given my heart to Jesus. Jacky told me on her walk they all prayed for her, and funny sounds came out of her mouth. The others had said it was the prayer language, *talking in other tongues* that only angels and God could understand. Although it felt supernaturally right, we both didn't understand a lot of it. But God had shown us He was real, He loved us both, and that was the best understanding of all.

When I arrived home and burst through the front door, you can imagine what Mother thought when I started saying I had talked to Jesus at the end of my bed – that I loved Him – and whatever He wanted me to do for my life – I would do it! I was in such an excited frenzy; Mother feared a religious sect had brainwashed me. No one behaved like this in the Uniting Church. The more I fired up about Jesus this – and Jesus that – the more she became increasingly concerned. I wasn't allowed to go back to the youth group. In my protective parents' view, I was behaving like someone being dragged naïvely into a cult, and they wouldn't let that happen. Desperate to keep my parents happy, I stopped going, and because I did, so did Jacky.

It didn't take long, and my youth group encounter with Jesus became a faded, distant memory. I became dragged down again very quickly with anxiety and fears over every little thing that entered my mind. My obsessive self-hate was alive and well and rose back up inside me in plague proportions. My faithful friend, alcohol, was waiting patiently for me, ready to numb my inner torment, and I soon began to drink secretly at home once more.

I left secondary school and studied at a business college. I excelled at typing and shorthand. Eventually, I was employed in an office and started earning an income. I was growing up and maturing, but unfortunately, emotionally I hadn't developed, and inside I was still a timid little girl. Graham was hardly ever home these days to push me around. My daily war-zone was less intense, and I was extremely grateful for the lengths of calm in my own home.

Over the next few years, Jacky and I had maintained our friendship. I was now 17, and she was 20. Our dynamic had not changed. Jacky emotionally ate for comfort while I drank, and we were still on the lookout to meet boys and have fun. Those two things were on the top of our list.

Jacky's older group of friends invited us to the German Club. I decided making my way into the party scene was what I needed to distract me from my negative inner voices which harassed me daily.

Anyway, the German Club sounded thrilling. I could wear make-up, get dressed up, drink alcohol, and dance. These are great ploys for getting a boy's attention. I needed to find a boyfriend. I needed to be loved to fill my unhappy void.

It was Friday night, and I was ready! Jacky's friends were picking me up at eight o'clock. I was so excited, and I couldn't wait to see what the night held for me.

CHAPTER 6

Desperate for Love

Getting drunk at the German Club was now a frequent Friday event. None of the boys at the youth group were interested in me, but the attention I got here as I circulated through the crowd was exciting!

I studied the German language at high school at an elementary level, so my parents were satisfied that I was going to the multicultural club for education purposes, which was half right. I knew *Wo ist Monica?* (Where is Monica?) and *Ist die post offen Otto?* (Is the post office open Otto?) Very handy! Never-the-less, Jacky and I slapped our knees with the buff German dancers and giggled at their little leather shorts and green felt hats covered in badges and feathers. We ate, *der brot und der franks*, and it was here I tasted my first black Russian. Vodka, Kahlua, and coke. Another medicinal recipe! It was sweet and bubbly and boosted my shy, low self-esteem with false confidence. Eleven years of Graham's constant put-downs – certainly helped evolve – my unhealthy view of myself. I desperately wanted to fit in, and I would do *anything* for that to be possible.

I wasn't the legal age to enter licensed premises, but no one ever asked me how old I was, so who would know? With a fancy dress, high heel shoes and a face dusted with makeup – I appeared very mature. Mother and Dad allowed me to go with Jacky and her friends, some who were in their late 20's. I felt very fashionable. I wanted to do everything they did, and of course, they encouraged me.

It was here at the German Club I met Jake Anderson. It was an instant attraction for both of us. He was Scottish, and his strong accent mesmerised me. Reasonably short and stocky, Jake had sandy hair, blue eyes, and a suntanned, well-built, muscular body. As a bricklayer by trade; you would expect nothing less than a fit physique. I was so shy and awkward – BUT – *A boy liked me!*

Being with him made me insecure and anxious. My obsessive thoughts drove me crazy. *Does he think I'm pretty? Will he like me? What if he doesn't like me?* It didn't matter what I did in my life; I was always anxious about it. I would obsess all day about little things, for example, *what colour nail polish would I paint my nails? Was it going to match what I would wear? What was I going to wear? Will Jake like me better in a dress or jeans? Do I look fat in jeans?* By the time I was ready to go out, I had spun myself into a tight knot. Then, I looked in the mirror and saw a girl who was never good enough, never pretty enough, and never deserving of anything.

But – good old alcohol was faithfully there – and always just a sip away. It numbed anxiety's tight grip on me.

I met Jake every Friday night at the German Club. When I saw him, his eyes twinkled in my direction, and my heart skipped a beat. He asked me to dance; I said yes. He asked me to be his girlfriend. I said, yes. Everything Jake asked me to do, I said yes. I was desperate for love – and I would do *anything*.

Jake asked me out on a surprise first date. He took me to the local drive-in theatre in his panel van. It was all decked out in the back with a mattress and a sound system. I felt so sassy at 17 to have a boyfriend with such a cool car.

Of course, his motive wasn't to watch a movie. I was so nervous and worried about having our first kiss, but Jake was planning far more than that. He wanted my virginity. I was an innocent lamb led to the slaughter.

Sex was a taboo subject in our home. Mother and Dad never talked about such things with me. At the Ladies College, we had sex-education lessons, but the teachers talked more about getting to know your own body, rather than having a baby. I was never one hundred percent sure of how it worked. I knew sex was sex, but to have a baby, I thought you had to do *something else* as well as sex to fall pregnant. You may think I was naïve, but I honestly thought I was not able to fall pregnant just by having sex. Jake reassured me I wouldn't, and I believed him. We used no protection. You didn't in those days. Parents never talked about such things with their children, and your friends with great excitement just wanted to know – "*Did you end up doing it?*"

It only happened once in the back of Jake's car that night – but once was enough. Then nearly two months later, I was holding in my hands, a piece of paper from the local pharmacy – confirming I was pregnant.

My parents, of course, were shocked and devastated when I told them. I told Mother first. With no expression, looking straight ahead, she stoically reassured me they would take care of everything. I wasn't sure what that meant. They discussed nothing with me. The next morning, I walked into my parent's bedroom, and I saw Dad cradled in Mother's arms sobbing. I knew it was because of what I had done. He looked up and spluttered words of disgust and anguish straight at me.

"*You are lower than an alley cat, screaming out in the gutter, and you are just like your birth mother. You are not of our blood! What else could we expect.*" Dad could hardly speak; he was crying so profoundly.

Yes, his words were harsh – though in essence – they were right. I ran back into my room, threw myself onto my bed, and cried into my pillow of a broken heart – because I had just broken Dads. I had never seen him cry before, and now in an instant, I was no longer Daddy's little girl. Knowing I had made him cry hurt me more than words can say. I was so sorry. Mother and Dad made all the arrangements for an abortion without discussing anything with me. In the meantime, I was grounded and forbidden to wear tight jeans ever again.

My parents allowed me to make one last phone call to Jake. As I dialled his number, I immediately felt sick. After a few rings, he picked up.

"Jake, it's Emma, how are you?" my voice was shaky.

"I'm good, Emma, what's up?" he replied.

"I have to tell you something, something big."
"Okay. What is it?"
"I've found out something."
"Okay! Just tell me!"
I could sense he was getting annoyed with me.
"I'm pregnant."
I started crying. Releasing this was too much for me.
"What the…?"
He sounded stunned.

I pleaded with him. "Jake, I want to keep it, but Mother and Dad say I have to have an abortion! I don't want an abortion."

I hoped he would say something like he loved me with an undying love, and we could run away together and live happily ever after!

I pleaded with him again, "Jake, I want to have this baby."
"Well, I don't want to have a kid."
He was cold and distant.
"You said you loved me, Jake."
He replied with, "How do I even know the kid's mine?"
He had no intention of taking any responsibility.
"Jake, you are my first," I whispered.
He stated coldly, "It's not my problem, Emma," and promptly hung up.

I never heard from him again.

I didn't want an abortion. I desperately wanted to keep my baby. I had no idea who my blood-line was. There was just me – all alone in this world not biologically connected to anybody. For the first time in my life, I had a person who was part of my flesh and blood. A person I could relate to and finally share an identity within this world. And this person was growing inside of me.

This child would connect me to our human race. I wouldn't feel like a lone island anymore. I wanted this more than anything. I sensed the baby was a boy, and I called him Paris, but no one knew I had called him this. Mother and Dad had arranged the abortion, and I couldn't do anything to stop it. I ached, in every part of my being, because this human life I desperately wanted to hold in my arms would never be mine. I stopped drinking at home as I knew this was bad for the baby, not that my decision had any long-term purpose for the child.

Day after day, I lay on my bed at home, limp and depressed. But no matter how much I pleaded with my parents to keep my baby, the gynaecologist procedure was fixed. I begged the doctor at one of my appointments to cancel everything, but he had no authority.

At 17, I was still under the legal care of my mother and father, and they were making the decision they saw best. I had no power to save my baby from its short-lived destiny.

Adoption wasn't commonplace anymore as it was in my mother's era in the 1960s. Abortions were now becoming increasingly popular.

It was the late 1970s, and the stigma of falling pregnant outside of marriage was still considered shameful. *Second-hand goods* was the term thrown around for any girl found in this situation, and the family name automatically suffered a hint of disgrace.

Abortions were now safer, more accessible, and a quick and non-disruptive operation. It only required a signature on a piece of paper, a day in the hospital, and then everyone's lives could carry on as usual without the black mark etched into the family line.

Even though abortions were slowly becoming a convenient form of birth control – we didn't know of anyone who had one – nor would anyone know about mine. Mother and Dad reassured me they were doing what was best for my future.

After one last invasive gynaecology check-up, the day arrived for me to pack my necessities and prepare myself for my hospital appointment. Dad drove me there on his way to work. The car ride seemed to take forever, with not a spoken word between us. As I sat silently in the back-seat, shame consumed me. *How bad I had been – how disgusting I was – how I had let everybody down.*

Dad stopped the car and sat still in his seat. That was my silent cue to get out. Without a goodbye, I walked up a cold, grey, lonely path towards the entrance doors of an old house now turned into a clinic. I carried two things: my small suitcase, and the little, innocent life growing inside me.

As I walked, I felt my baby's flutters. Not that the doctors were counting, or cared, but I was just over four months pregnant. I laid my hands on my stomach and whispered, "I'm so sorry, Paris, my darling baby, please forgive me."

I was nauseous with grief. I wanted to run. Run anywhere and to anyone who could help me keep my baby, but I had no idea where to go for help. Knowing an imminent death sentence was organised for this baby with every step I took made me sick to my core.

I pushed open the large, white, heavy wooden door. There was no reception area. No one came to see if I needed any assistance. I didn't know what to do, where to go, or what to say.

I just stood there feeling helpless and alone.

A nurse walked towards me. Trying to make eye contact, I blurted out, "Excuse me; I have an appointment for today!" She looked at me, appeared extremely annoyed, pointed her finger sharply and barked her command as if I was a dog, "Sit down there and wait!" Of course, I obeyed promptly.

I sat still and silent, for an hour to be exact. It felt like an eternity. Because I was only 17, I needed my guardian's signature on my admission slip. That detail somehow got missed along the way. Dad had to drive back to the clinic from work and sign the legal papers. This oversight made everyone involved even more annoyed.

Another nurse came and gave me a heavy steel bedpan and a white cotton gown without any instruction. She led me into one of the rooms, walked out, and shut the door. No one talked to me, and I felt like a naughty little girl. I assumed they wanted a urine sample. Or was this in case I felt like vomiting? Because I did.

I looked around the room. It resembled a bedroom in the pioneer days. There was one old-fashioned metal single bed, an old chest of drawers, and a dark, brown wooden wardrobe – which I instantly hated.

The room was dim and sterile. Where was the toilet? Do I just squat in the middle of the room to fill this pan? I was so shy and embarrassed in case someone walked in.

I knew I would get growled at if I didn't supply a sample, so carrying the heavy bedpan, I went over to the wardrobe and climbed up inside, leaving the door open just a crack for fresh air. As much as I feared wardrobes, I had no other option for privacy. Being inside instantly gave me an anxiety rush. It was dark and musty. I started to cry. The flutters of my baby were soft and gentle, as I held the pan in between my semi-bent legs.

Choking back my emotion, I whispered, "I'm sorry Paris, I'm so sorry!"

My skin tingled, and a shiver ran up my back. Someone had just stepped over my grave, and I had an eerie projection of déjà vu. I pondered for a moment to see if anything familiar came to me. No, nothing. Whatever it was, it certainly wasn't pleasant. I couldn't wait to get out, which I must say took very talented balancing skills holding the semi-full, heavy, large metal pan. I had fulfilled the nurse's unspoken request with regret. I wanted to be anywhere else but here.

I left the bedpan on the chest of drawers, put on the hospital gown, and got into the bed. Finally, another mute nurse came and gave me an anaesthetic, while I lay on the cold linen sheets. This room had no warmth, and the nurses had no personality. I sensed they were angry with me for being there. I was angry with myself, too.

Within minutes I became sleepy. My eyelids were getting heavy, but I remember someone wheeling me into the operating theatre, where the doctor introduced himself to me. Why on earth would I want to meet the man who is going to kill my baby?

With a smile on his face, he said, "You'll be asleep in a couple of minutes." Inside I screamed at him. My thoughts raced in a confused, suppressed rage.

"Is this fun for you? Do you love your job, killing innocent unborn babies? Aren't you glad your mother didn't have an abortion? I hate you, I…h…a…t…e…y…"

The next thing I knew, I was awake, back in my room laying in the hospital bed. The anaesthetic had worn off, and my mouth was dry. My stomach was tender. I was empty, and without invitation, grief settled upon me.

My baby was gone. The warmth and flutters I had felt just hours ago were not there anymore. I could feel that Paris had been scraped away from inside me. The loss was unbearable. He was my only connection to this world I lived in, and now he was gone. I ached in every part of my being.

Later that afternoon, Mother came to the hospital and picked me up. I sensed she was glad it was all over. It was another silent car ride home, and this ordeal was never to be spoken of again.

I tried to put it all behind me as best I could. Grief overpowered any happiness I had in my life. Guilt plagued my thoughts. How could I have been responsible for such a thing? *I killed my baby.*

I blamed and hated myself for that. My self-esteem dropped down further than it had ever been. I felt uglier than I had ever felt.

Anxiety now pulsed through me all the time, and I felt so far away from God. I never prayed anymore. How could God ever forgive me for killing my baby? I was lost and desperate to know who I was. My life was a continual black hole and seemingly hopeless.

My soul-searching quest for the meaning of my life was fast becoming an insatiable cry. *I needed to know who I was, where I came from, and what my purpose was here on earth.*

Two girls from my work – Pippa and Sally – were talking about having their tarot cards read. Pippa knew of a white witch who told futures, and she had a reputation for being very accurate. I keenly jumped on board. Maybe someone could tell me if there was any hope ahead for me.

CHAPTER 7

Unforetold Future

Pippa, Sally, and I set off straight after work as planned. We drove to a little weatherboard house out in a commercial zone. There were no other houses around, only factories. I immediately conjured up thoughts; it was a haunted house, and no one would ever see us again!

I didn't tell Mother and Dad what I was doing, as this fiercely went against my Methodist Church upbringing. I definitely wouldn't be allowed to be involved in anything of this nature.

Pippa pulled up slowly into the driveway. We all sat quietly in the car.

"This feels spooky!" I said.

"Oh, Em, don't be silly." Pippa piped up. "It's just a bit of fun!"

"Yes, but spooky fun," I said with a worried frown.

We all laughed.

"What time was our appointment?" I asked.

"We don't have one," Sally said.

"What?" I panicked. "She might be angry; we have disturbed her!"

I had been uneasy about this all day, and now we had arrived, I was extremely anxious. Pippa put on her best ghoulish voice and mystically moved her hands, trying to scare us all.

"The witch might grab us and lock us in her dungeon; fatten us up, and eat us, one by one!"

"Stop it, Pip." I smacked her arm. "You know I scare easily!"

Sally asked, "Who is going to be brave enough to knock on the door?"

Sally and I both voted for Pip. The house was small and surrounded by bushes and trees, as though it was hiding. We strolled up a grey concrete path until we reached the front door. Pippa clenched her fist and gave a few quick bangs. The front veranda welcomed us with an eeriness. Then we all stood very still and just waited. After a little while, the door opened slowly. A tall, slim lady with long, black hair appeared, wearing a red velvet gown. She seemed a bit dishevelled, as though she had just thrown on her dress, but very quickly, she gathered herself and put on a polite smile for us.

"Can I help you?" she spoke softly.

Her mystical presence was noticeable and quite intimidating.

Sally spoke up. "We wondered…if you could tell us our futures?"

Through stony eyes and rigid body language, we could tell she was not delighted the three of us had come.

She looked out the front door – to the left and the right – suspicious we had perhaps brought the police with us. It was widely considered fortune-tellers worked illegally and were seen as purely taking money from desperate people. Their occult talents were considered hocus pocus, and even dangerous by many. They were not at all held in high regard. The consensus was to avoid coming to such practices.

She replied in a monotone, trying to brush us off. "No, not today, I'm tired. Your readings might not be accurate."

Immediately, the three of us whined. We told the witch we had driven a long way, and it would be impossible for the three of us to all come together again at the same time. We pleaded with her, and very annoyed, she ushered us in – more to keep us quiet than anything else.

"It's going to be $15 each. My name is Esmeralda, and you can come into this room here," her arm theatrically waving towards us.

We all nodded and followed – almost in a trance. The room was dim and a little bit dusty. A medieval atmosphere of candles and numerous ornaments of the dark side, such as dragons, towers, skulls, and snakes, were on display all around the room.

A medium-sized round table covered with a purple velvet cloth blended beautifully with five ornate, tapestry upholstered chairs. Placed around the table in a perfect semi-circle, I felt a distinct sense; the chairs contained a dark power of their own. It was as though they were awaiting our arrival for spiritual activity.

The hairs on my back stood up. I felt a presence that made me very uncomfortable. Pippa, Sally, and I awkwardly sat down. Esmeralda walked over to a side cabinet and brought back a large deck of cards.

"She certainly looks the part!" Pippa whispered, and all our eyes widened.

"Shhhhh!" I breathed out gently.

I'm sure Esmerelda heard that comment and was not impressed. We had entered her realm of mastery, one of which she took very seriously. One by one, we had a turn, and Pippa and Sally were happy with their predicted futures. When it came to me, Esmeralda said she had a headache and felt a bit fuzzy. I pressured her to consider the unfairness of leaving me out. She let out a huge sigh of annoyance and reluctantly shuffled the cards.

Before she lay anything down on the table, she asked, "Do you have a brother?"

I replied, "Yes."

She pondered this for a second and then started placing cards down in front of me.

She turned over the death and tower card, and quite a few other sinister-looking cards as well. She stared at them with no expression. She exhaled a few more breaths and appeared stuck. Then she screwed up her face and commented that a light so bright was shining into her eyes; it stopped her seeing any more. Now she was very irritated. She stood to her feet. The reading was over.

I left feeling the odd one out. *Why don't I seem to fit in anywhere; who am I and where am I heading in this life?* Even the white witch didn't know. I felt even more frustrated and confused, but I would never give up my pursuit of love and happiness, and so I kept going out to the pubs with high hopes.

Unexpectedly, one night out at our local hotel, I met Bruce, and he became my boyfriend. He was an adorable person and treated me like a princess. He would have given me the world. Do you know what I did? I sabotaged the relationship and ended it.

My self-esteem was so low; I convinced myself I wasn't good enough for him. My self-hate was so high; I didn't deserve anyone to treat me so wonderfully.

His adoration felt uncomfortable and foreign to me. I was used to being poorly treated. Having someone respect me, and be kind and gentle with me was strange, and I wasn't worthy of a love like this.

I was unaware of the severe and permanent damage Graham had inflicted on my subconscious over the years. My scars were internal, and though invisible, they were there, and deeply buried. I told myself that Bruce deserved someone much better than me. I did him a favour by breaking up with him. Now he could find someone better.

What you believe, you receive – and that left me in a lot of trouble.

After a couple more years of dating, I realised I attracted a type. The bad boy type. The arrogant men who are full of charisma, totally conceited, and naturally selfish in every way. They treated me in the way I felt I deserved. They put me second in the relationship, jeered at my faults, put me down in public, and dominated me into submission.

My automatic reaction always centred around pleasing them – and them only. And I did it so well. It came naturally for me. I felt comfortable doing this, and so long as this dynamic played out between us, the relationship went very smoothly. Of course, my rewards were empty promises and dangled carrots that never came, but I was forever hopeful.

CHAPTER 8

Is Someone Looking out for Me?

At 19 years of age and permeated with the side-effects of alcohol, I lived recklessly.

My little girl inside was broken, and my search to find *anyone* to fix her was my subconscious agenda.

Internally fragmented, two identities were living inside me. A frightened little girl who was crying out for healing, and a damaged woman; standing on a shaky emotional foundation, lost, broken, and vulnerable.

Each had nothing to offer the other. Each would cry out for a reconciliation of the soul, but the chasm between them was dark and vast. The two hearts never spoke. They gave one another no advice, nurture, or self-love. The two were miles apart and utterly alone.

For me to be whole, healing must take place between my little girl and my woman. Until then, I was in a dangerous situation because I lived with a damaged little girl's mentality and perspective of life, in a grown-up world, and all my woman could do was stand back helplessly and watch from a distance.

One night, my new girlfriend, Jessie, and I drove home from a night out at the clubs. It was now the early hours of the morning, and the streets were like a ghost town. I was the nominated driver that night, but that didn't mean anything. I would always drink and drive.

Approaching a red light, I slowed down. It was only 30 seconds or so, and another car pulled up beside us. Two guys greeted us with flashy smiles. Responding with giggles of invitation, the flirting had begun.

The other driver revved his engine. I acknowledged his advances and revved mine. The drag race was on. Our cars entwined together to roaring sounds filling the atmosphere, waiting for the traffic light to turn green.

His car roared off at high speed while I got off to a slow start, with billowing smoke surrounding my vehicle. In my drunken state, I had inadvertently left on the hand-brake. I had now blown the gearbox, and Jessie and I were not going anywhere.

Like damsels in distress, we waited for our knights in shining armour to return gallantly to rescue us, and sure enough, they did.

I locked my car, and without thinking, Jessie and I climbed into the backseat of their two-door hatchback.

As we sat still in the back, Jessie and I looked at each and realised we were now trapped. What had we done? We didn't know who these guys were, and we had no door to escape.

"How's your night been girls?" the driver asked.

My whole body rushed with panic. I looked at Jessie, and from the expression she gave me, I knew she felt the same.

"Good," I answered shyly.

Jessie spoke up, "Can you give us a lift home, please?"

Silence.

Suddenly I was scared, and it was apparent to both of us we were now in trouble. I sobered up almost instantly.

The guy driving said to his mate, "Hey, which one do you want? I think I am going to go with the tall skinny one. She looks like she wants some."

Jessie was quite short, so that meant me. My heart raced, and my whole body went into high danger alert mode. I couldn't think of what we could do.

Jessie spoke again, "Um, we are tired, and we would be very grateful if you could take us home."

Again, no response. I looked at Jessie in sheer panic. All I could think of was to pray.

Internally, I screamed towards heaven. *Please, please, please, God, HELP US! I beg you. Keep us safe.*

There was more silence, the only interaction being an occasional glance back at us, followed by a sinister smirk. The atmosphere was pure evil. I fervently continued my silent petitions to God.

After a short while, out of the blue, the driver spoke to his mate. "Hey buddy, I am not feeling it. I've got a bit of a headache coming on. Might give this one a miss tonight!"

Buddy replied with a smirk, "Yeah, cool dude, no worries. There will be other times, for sure!"

The driver's eyes penetrated right through me from the rear vision mirror. "Yeah girls, what's your address, we will drop you off."

My heart sank with gratefulness. With a shallow breath, I managed to tell the driver the name of the street before mine. Jessie and I could walk a block to get home. There was no way I was going to let him know where my house was. With heightened anticipation, we sat quietly with the promise we were going to be safe.

As Jessie and I scrambled out of the two-door hatch, we shouted our thank you on the run. Getting as far away from them was our only focus. As I watched the car drive away, I looked up at the night sky twinkling with stars and couldn't help but wonder; is someone looking out for me?

CHAPTER 9

Overflowing with Charisma

My parents organised a European holiday and insisted I travel with them. I sensed they knew how sad I was with life, and this was their way of trying to help. They hoped this experience would give me a fresh outlook to see that the world is a big and beautiful place full of exciting opportunities.

On our Italian tour, I met an Australian girl named Brittany, who lived in Melbourne. She was a very striking, olive-skinned, slim brunette. Brittany looked Italian herself. At 25 years of age and working in the tourism industry, she was well-travelled and experienced in the ways of the world. There was an aura of destiny surrounding our meeting, and we both had a sense of excitement to see where our friendship would take us after our holiday.

My parents immediately didn't like her, but my parents didn't approve of anyone I attracted. I always thought it was the generation gap between them and me, and they were just old fuddy-duddies. So, I never heeded their wisdom. At 19, I knew it all!

When our Italian tour came to an end, Brittney and I swapped numbers and vowed to catch up. It was only a few weeks later when I heard from her. Brittany had organised a job transfer from Melbourne to the Gold Coast. She invited me to relocate too and share an apartment with her. I couldn't think of anything more thrilling! An exciting opportunity had presented itself to me, and I was all in, despite my parent's concerns.

This move wasn't permanent. I planned to have a 12-month working holiday. Grandma and I were still best friends, and I made a promise to her I would be home for Christmas day. Christmas was sacred in our family. I left my job, sold my car, and within a few weeks, I arrived on the Coast.

Brittany's apartment was gorgeous. The high-rise towered over the beach with views right out of a travel magazine. We swam, sun-baked, shopped, and drove around town in her snazzy little powder-blue 911 Porsche Carrera Cabriolet convertible. Two new 'It Girls' had arrived on the scene, and soon we were turning heads. I loved all the attention. We transitioned quickly into the Gold Coast lifestyle. I found a job as a receptionist at a successful Law firm, and Brittany and I flowed beautifully together in our cosmopolitan way of living.

It wasn't long before we were strutting our stuff at the nightclub – *The Pink Flamingo*. It was the socialite place to be after dark. We became members of the club and very quickly earned our place of popularity amongst the locals. Back in the 1980s, Surfers Paradise was the trendiest place to be in Australia. Finally, I fitted in somewhere.

Every night the Flamingo was buzzing with people, and this particular Saturday night was no exception. Locals gathered in their usual huddles, sprinkled with a few apparent tourists. Disco lights flickered upon tanned, fit bodies, hoping everyone would notice their stylish moves. And then I saw him – and he saw me! Our eyes locked, and yes, it was one of those surreal, across a crowded room, moments.

He walked straight over to me and introduced himself as Andrew. I responded with a polite handshake, and he grabbed my hand and pulled me onto the dance floor. All night long, we danced, flirted, and sipped cocktails. After scribbling my phone number on the corner of a napkin, I floated all the way home, hoping I would see him again soon. Of course, I did, and it wasn't long before we were officially Gold Coast's newest item.

Brittany became insanely jealous. Her reaction towards me finding a boyfriend was not the excited; *I am happy for you, girlfriend!* She promptly told me I belonged to her and her only and forbid me to see

Andrew. I suspected she might have been bi-sexual although she had never tried anything on me.

In her disappointed rage, she flushed all my belongings down the rubbish chute and sink disposal. I had to escape the apartment with a secret, quick exit, and the few things I had left. Mother and Dad were right in their perceptions about her. I found a room to rent close to where Andrew lived and settled into the Gold Coast life with him.

Incredibly good looking, Andrew oozed charisma. Sun-bleached blonde hair, naturally paired with his tanned, muscular body, and of course a beach-white smile. A real Surfers Paradise local boy. You could always find him during the day at the beach riding the waves.

Andrew said he liked me because I wasn't like all the other superficial girls on the Coast – even though I was trying very hard to be. Andrew said many times he had never met anyone like me before. I never knew if this was a compliment or not, but Andrew had chosen to be with ME! We had so much fun together, and I shared everything with him except one thing – the inadequacy I felt to be his girlfriend.

Most of the girls on the Gold Coast came here to find *sugar-daddies* and the older, wealthy men were always on the hunt for a new fresh little thing to boost their egos. It wasn't long before I had an offer for riches and trinkets from an extremely well-to-do French man who was in partnership with my bosses. His name was Jacques, and he found a reason to visit our office every day. It was business; personal business – it was to see *me!*

Jacques' temptations consisted of jewellery, perfume, and an unlimited credit card. He offered to set me up in a unit, buy me a brand-new Mercedes – and I never had to work again! Of course, there was a fine print clause – regular, private company with him. Jacques was old enough to be my father! For me, it was wrong on so many levels! Besides, Andrew captivated me.

Our relationship was young and exciting, but because of my old patterns of low self-worth, it didn't take long before I took my place as the insecure, dating doormat.

Soon everything centred around what Andrew wanted, and I was too timid to stand up for myself. He pressured me to do some modelling. He was signed up to a local magazine and had contacts to get me some work too. But the thought of competing with the long-legged Gold Coast beauties increased my anxiety. I couldn't do it!

Then it started. Andrew insisted I have a model look, *all the time*. He expressed, if I lost some weight, grew my hair longer, worked on my tan, I would be *more* attractive! I might add here, I wasn't fat, but Andrew made continual remarks about me being frumpy and unappealing. He tapped my thighs or chin when we walked past a girl boasting model-like qualities, which on the Gold Coast, is all the time.

I could never reach Andrew's high expectations, no matter what I did. I just wanted him to value me for who I was, but that was never going to happen.

He introduced me to marijuana. I hadn't tried it before, and I didn't like it, but I smoked it anyway, just in case he broke up with me. I drank too much; I smoked too much. I worried too much. My life was spiralling out of control, and our relationship appeared to be going nowhere. I didn't have any long-term goals or plans with him. Andrew was indifferent about our relationship and didn't seem upset that one day I would be going home. Eventually, the year was up, and the time came for me to return to the West. Once again, I felt chewed up and spat out. With a broken heart, I said goodbye to the beautiful Gold Coast and Andrew.

I settled back into Perth. All my friends were glad I was home, and I found a new job. I missed Andrew terribly and tried to put the last year behind me.

To my surprise, Andrew tracked me down, sprouting sonnets that he couldn't live without me. He packed up his life on the Gold Coast and moved over to the West. He asked me to marry him, and I ecstatically said, *yes!* Did I love Andrew? I loved the fact *somebody* wanted me, and *somebody* wanted to marry me. I loved that I wasn't rejected and that I wouldn't be on my own and alone.

All my life, I had longed for my Cinderella fairy tale. I craved for my prince to show up, take me in his arms and dance with me forever. Now, Andrew and I would live happily ever after.

So, I waited for the ring. After a long time, Andrew finally shared his delay with me. It went like this. In 20 years, when I'd be 40, if I was fat, he didn't know if he could love me! To be clear, I wasn't fat. I was 20, toned and trim. I was often complimented on my petite figure. But Andrew's fear of me getting fat in my later years was real for him. So real, he broke up with me.

I was devastated.

My self-hate increased, and my low self-esteem skyrocketed. Then we did a yo-yo act. Andrew pleaded with me to take him back as he couldn't live without me. So, I took him back – only to go through the same scenario of a marriage proposal and becoming fat when I'm 40 – three more times over two years.

After two years of enduring Andrew's topsy-turvy love for me, I was heartbroken and angry. Psychologically this had affected me more than anyone realised. I became determined – *never to get fat* – EVER! And certainly not when I'm 40. So, an internal war against myself to always be thin began.

The insipid, slithering voice I was only too familiar with all my life now had new ammunition to whisper in my ear.

Don't get fat! You are so ugly anyway; you will be even more obnoxious if you get fat! And then NO ONE will EVER love you!

Day after day, as I looked in the mirror, it reflected an image that convinced me my thoughts were right. I had a distorted view of myself through a lens of fear. Fear I would never be good enough for this world – nor anybody – not even myself. I hated myself with such a passion. Every day, I became obsessed with strategies of how I could become thinner. It consumed every waking moment in my thoughts. I believed this voice because this was the only voice I heard. *I was fat, and I was ugly.*

Food became my enemy instead of a sustaining friend. I was paranoid about letting calories enter my body, and I believed the only way to be accepted and beautiful was if I was thin. A world dictated continuously; I was not appealing, sexy, attractive, or lovable – if I was not skinny. And it was true. See, Andrew didn't want me for all these reasons.

But the truth was – I hadn't accepted myself. I believed others saw me on the outside, how I felt about myself on the inside. Ugly and unlovable! I kept losing weight, but no matter how much I lost, I always saw myself – as fat.

I didn't know at 22 years of age; I had invited a disease into my life called anorexia. I was severely nutrient deficient. My body mass index was four, and I had zero fat on my body. Although I kept drinking alcohol, I made up for the calories by starving myself at every meal, and eventually, my monthly cycle stopped. At five feet, eight inches, I was a baggy size six in my clothes, and I weighed 47 kilos. I wouldn't even drink water for fear of retaining fluid. But no matter what my efforts were to be thin, when I looked in the mirror – I was always fat.

Andrew stalked me for a year, pleading with me to get back with him. My answer was no, though knowing he was spying on me gave me an incentive to lose more inches to prove to him I would never be fat at 40. Eventually, he gave up, but I didn't. I formed one insatiable, all-consuming goal for my life. A goal never to eat.

It took a couple of agonising years, with the help of my loving and supportive parents, to get my mind and body back to normality and out of the grip of anorexia. Then I developed *bulimia*. I would gorge myself on food because I was so hungry. I was never the vomiting kind, so I would starve myself for three to five days, depending on how much I had eaten. This pattern of gorging and denying myself food lasted about a year. It took Mother and Dad round the clock dedication and patience to help me break this mental habit and ease me back into healthy eating. Even to this day – 35 years later – I will always give thought to what I put into my body and if it will make me fat. I eat clean and have the odd treat. I certainly enjoy food now, but I'm not sure if the faint, haunting voices will ever leave.

I was able to keep the diseases under control, but not the fear monster in my mind, which tormented me daily with negative thoughts about my self-image. I might not have been fat, but I was still ugly. I continued to numb my subconscious and vile pestering with my old faithful friend alcohol which I drank every day, although my parents didn't know. I was able to function and hold down a job, but appearances are very deceptive. We can learn very quickly what masks to wear, and we wear them well to cover up what we don't want others to see.

Two people in my life passed away that year. The first was Jacky. She committed suicide. I had been to her wedding a few years earlier, and everything seemed beautiful. It was lovely to see Jacky had finally accepted herself. She had gone back to church and met a kind man who loved her for just being – Jacky. She had found a love to help her diffuse her internal ticking time-bomb. Or so we all thought. She wore her mask of happiness well. No one had any idea how desperate she must have been. A passer-by found Jacky in the bush in her car. She had hooked up the exhaust to come through the window and died of gas poisoning.

It was such a shock for everyone, but not really for me. I probably knew Jacky better than anyone. She and her husband had been arguing, but it hadn't appeared to be that bad. Sometimes, just one little thing in your life can be the straw that breaks the camel's back.

Jacky had years of suppressed misery because of rejection and self-hate.

I understood. Jacky was too tired to fight her black hole of sadness anymore. Two weeks later, her husband was found deceased in the same car, in the same spot, in the same bush. He had gassed himself as well. It was a double tragedy, beyond tragedies.

Hopelessness and despair are not something to be ashamed of or covered up with a false mask. Compassion and understanding are what we need for anyone with depression and mental illness. We promote that not reaching out for help is the problem. And while this is true –

there is also another just as dangerous – the problem of hiding it so well.

My darling Grandma also passed away in her sleep at the age of 87. The night before she died, her face appeared to me in a dream. She said, *I love you, Emma*, and I replied, *I love you, Grandma*. We embraced and said goodbye to each other.

When Mother rang me the next day and told me of her passing, it wasn't a shock. In my heart, I knew she had passed away. My Grandma had gone, and I missed her dearly, but I keep her close in my affections. She left me her wedding ring as promised, and it is my valued possession. Not for any monetary gain, but for the deep love connection we shared.

After losing two exceptional people, I was in a low place. There were not too many highlights in my life after that, though I was happy in my job. I worked in a Government office for the Minister for Police, and although it was a nine to five mundane atmosphere, it was reassuring that my position was secure.

Being trained on the typewriter was a great skill to have, and my speed was efficient, but a new sleek machine was coming onto the market to promote the workload being accomplished even faster. It was called *the computer*, and all the government offices were switching over. In Western Australia, we were the first offered this system, and all the girls underwent immediate training to operate these fast and flashy devices.

And they were fast. We sat at our desks, fingers tapping at triple the pace, churning out triple the workload. The bosses were ecstatic, and we felt proud of their praises.

A few girls started to complain of a burning sensation in their forearms, but this was overlooked and not taken seriously. The efficiency of the workload was more crucial. Then one day after work catching the bus home, my arms became heavy. I couldn't open my purse to pay the bus driver. What was wrong with me? It was so embarrassing; I needed help. The ride home seemed to take forever and trapped me in a time-warp of pain. A burning sensation began prickling under the skin in my forearms.

By the time I arrived home, I was in complete distress. I couldn't turn the door key to enter my house. My arms felt like concrete. I had to knock and wait until Mother came and opened the door for me. Sharing with my parents what was happening to the other girls, and now myself, posed a dilemma. I had no choice but to report my condition, which was getting significantly worse, day by day.

I was placed in the *too hard basket* with all the other girls with sore arms. No one knew what was happening – least of all us. By the end of week two, my arms were a dead-weight, and the knife-stabbing pain burned as though a bush fire was raging out of control under my skin. It was relentless and wouldn't go away. I accepted a transfer to light duties, and I stopped typing. My boss was furious. The atmosphere in the office was one of disdain and frustration, as the other girls whose arms were not sore had to pick up our workload as well. It was a vicious circle. The more girls that were added to light duties, the faster the rest had to go. Soon, the too hard basket was full of girls with heavy and burning arms. Government investigators came to determine what this mysterious affliction was that was plaguing us.

Finally, it had a name. It was repetitive strain injury, otherwise known as RSI. We were all diagnosed with it and offered physiotherapy as a form of compensation for the damage, but this was no quick remedy. Repair was up to the individual, and time and rest were the only given healers. I was in excruciating agony 24/7 and no pain remedy slew it. I couldn't brush my teeth or hair, pick up a fork to eat, drive my car, or even fasten my bra. Everything I took for granted was now an impossibility. The Government Department allocated me 12 months of unpaid sick leave.

Recovery was going to be a long, slow road. Some friends of mine had moved to the United Kingdom, and I thought a complete change of country would do me a world of good, literally! The escape was not just to rest my arms, but also to clear my life from Andrew's toxic head games, and the grief I was experiencing from the loss of my loved ones.

They say culture broadens the mind and travel clears the cobwebs and this was just what I needed. In my travels I had numerous good times caught on film and made many amazing memories.

We all have funny stories that have happened to us that make other people laugh as well as ourselves.

Here are three of mine I would love to share when I went to visit my friends in England.

CHAPTER 10

Just for a Giggle

Through a London travel agent, I booked a three-week holiday around Europe with Top Deck Tours. They had a reputation for having wild adventures specifically for young people. A fun get-away was what I needed. Top Deck's fleet of buses were all painted yellow and orange and had names, like a family. Our bus was Gordon.

At our initial meet and greet instantly, I made 17 friends from all over the world. We were a mixed bunch of nationalities, and we knew we were all going to have loads of fun. There was a Singaporean born-again Christian, a Chinese Hindu, an American man, engaged New Zealanders' and the rest of us guys and gals were loud Aussies from all parts of Australia.

We received a list of personal items to bring, one of which was a sleeping bag. I was purposefully travelling in the middle of winter as I had always wanted to experience the joys of snow – a sleeping bag…hmmm. I hot-footed down to the local London camping store and perused all the padded cocoons for sale. Being a thrifty traveller, I bought the cheapest one. Some were two hundred pounds, and I wasn't going to spend that much when I could get one for ten. Besides, seasoned bus-tour-group-people had told me that the heaters on the bus keep you extremely warm and you don't need a thick one.

The exciting day came, and we all met at the White Cliffs of Dover to board the ferry to Amsterdam, our first starting point on our European route. Gordon was also there, full of fuel and ready to go. It was a quick trip across the channel, and by the time the ferry pulled into the Netherlands' dock, it was dark.

We all clambered into Gordon and found a seat, laughing and talking, creating an atmosphere of adventure. Gordon chugged along confidently as he had travelled along Amsterdam's cobbled roads many a time before.

Europe's air was ice cold. It might have been all right, except Gordon – who I think by the look of him was about 50-years-old – was falling apart, and his ancient heating system broke down on day one of our three-week winter wonderland trip. It was freezing! I had never experienced a cold like this ever before. When I say ice cold, I mean, *ice-cold!* And all I had was my ten-pound summer sleeping bag.

Well, I froze. No, listen, *I froze!* Literally! As did *everything!* At the end of every wet day, everyone draped their socks, scarves, and gloves over Gordon's seats hoping they would dry overnight. Everything we possessed was soaked.

We all slept on the floor of the bus down the middle aisle like sardines in a tin can. The night icy-air transformed Gordon into a cold storage container. Of course, everyone else had thick, warm, fluffy bedding, while I had the thinness of a sheet. In the morning, you could snap the socks in two; they were frozen stiff! I felt like I could snap in two as well. Even my camera froze in my bag. The spool of film stuck to the internal mechanisms and wouldn't wind on.

I paid my reluctant friends generously to zip our sleeping bags together so that I wouldn't die in the night of hypothermia. I could have bought ten, thick sleeping bags by the time our holiday was over!

The 21 snow-filled days of travel allowed us to capture many postcard countryside photographs. Majestic castles proudly boasted the rich, royal history of Germany. Metre-long icicles hung from log cabins with cosy fires in Switzerland. Romantic whispers heard throughout the streets of Paris added to the ambience of affection. Coins kissed with the hope of love eternal – one by one – were thrown into the Trevi Fountain in Rome. We ate delicious national dishes, drank different beers and wines, saw all the local tourist attractions, and bought plenty of keyrings and fridge magnets!

The snow was beautiful. Cold but beautiful! The holiday finally came to an end. I couldn't wait to get back to London and plan a warmer trip, so I ventured over to Greece for a short stay.

∼

My friends in England had a friend, of a friend, of a friend, named Costa, who lived in Greece on the coast of Crete. When you travel, these friendly hook-ups are not unusual. My friends kindly organised through Costa a place for me to stay and arranged some work for me through his business. It was bar work. I had never pulled a beer tap before or made fancy cocktails, though I always had a big smile, and I am a fast learner.

As soon as I arrived in Crete, I set out to find Costa's bar. Situated opposite a shipping port, many of the patrons were sailors and riggers. I was nervous and excited; feeling like the world was my oyster. I didn't know what a bar girl wore, so I dressed in a black skirt and a white blouse as I knew this was appropriate for hospitality.

I walked through the hotel doors, and although this establishment was small, it contained a warm and friendly atmosphere. There were a couple of girls sitting at the bar by themselves, and a few men at a table having a quiet drink together. Costa was awaiting my arrival, and greeted me with a flashy white smile, before smacking flamboyant kisses on my cheek.

Costa had a nice tan, and of course, was oozing with handsome European charm. His soft cream silk shirt and pale blue slacks teamed very nicely with the thick gold chain around his neck. He had a gold ring on nearly every finger and was continually running them through his long, greying hair. Costa would have been a stud in his day, and even now, was still a charmer with the women. He didn't speak English well, and I couldn't understand most of what he said, but he made me blush.

No one spoke English well, so I used hand gestures and smiled. Costa motioned for me to sit at the bar and wait. I politely obliged, becoming more nervous by the minute. I supposed when he was ready he would train me in how to serve the customers, who were mainly men and now starting to enter the pub in steady numbers.

I smiled at one of the girls a few times sitting at the bar, and she smiled back. She was pretty and wore a sparkly dress with high heel shoes. I assumed she must be waiting for her boyfriend to celebrate a special occasion. A couple of men started talking to me, and I chatted back, talking about my Europe escapades, Gordon's lack of heating, and my ten-pound sleeping bag. I kept a keen eye out for Costa. He was always distracted, talking and laughing with the patrons, and he seemed to have forgotten about me. I approached the pretty girl sitting at the bar to see if she knew any English. Maybe she could ask Costa what was going on with me working here.

"Hi, my name is Emma." I smiled and held out my hand.

With a strong accent, she replied, "I am Jacinta; it is nice to meet you here."

She shook my hand and asked me quite straightforwardly, "So, you are working for Costa too now?"

Thrilled she spoke English, I replied, "Um, yes, I start tonight. I'm so nervous! I have never worked in a bar before, or made a cocktail, and if my mother knew I was pulling on a beer tap in a pub, she would kill me, but I'm sure I will get the hang of it."

She smiled and responded, "I have been working here for two years now. Costa pays well, and there is always the extra if you want it!"

"Oh, cool!" I said.

I didn't quite understand what she meant by *the extra*, but I was sure as I got more skilled and experienced, Costa would promote me too.

I asked Jacinta curiously, "So, are you working tonight?" She wasn't dressed appropriately for serving behind the bar, and there didn't seem to be enough room for both of us.

She laughed at me, "What do you mean? I am working already. Just like you."

My mind went blank for a split second, "I don't understand, Jacinta."

She was frustrated by my comment and started cussing passionately in Greek to herself. Then she apologised. "Sorry, Emma, it's not your fault. It's just that this is not the first time Costa does not explain and leaves it up to me."

"What do you mean, Jacinta?" I was quite baffled.

"You see, Emma, you just sit at the bar. The men come in. You smile, you flirt. They buy you drinks. If you want to drink alcohol, say Scotch and coke or whatever you wish, and whoever is working behind the bar will pour that for you. If you don't want to drink alcohol, tell whoever is working beforehand you don't want to, but then say Scotch and coke, and he will give you coke but charges the man for Scotch and coke. Either way, Costa makes his profit. I find drinking too much alcohol every night gets too much, so if I want it, I wink, and if I don't, I don't wink."

"What?" I blurted out. "My job is to sit and drink and talk?"

Jacinta attempted to explain in her best English. "Mainly. But if you want more money, you can go home with a man and ask for money. You know – for the sex!"

"Oh!" I answered, shocked but trying to look like I wasn't. As desperate as I was for love, I knew travelling in a different country, I had to be careful.

A large group of raucous sailors had just entered, and instantly I felt like tempting bait for a pack of hungry dogs. A cute young sea-faring man with a perfectly-ironed white uniform approached me and asked if he could buy me a drink. Jacinta nodded at me, encouraging me with well wishes for my first customer.

"Um," I stuttered to the sailor, "Ouzo and coke, please."

I didn't tap or wink or nod toward the bartender. I needed a drink – and a *double* would be fantastic! I was still in shock from what Jacinta had just told me. After I composed myself with the reality that I was probably an escort; I chattered away quite nervously to all the patrons. I always had my sleeping bag and frozen camera story if conversation lagged.

After a few Ouzo and cokes, I was having a great time. Throughout my conversations, I let all the lads know, I would *not* be available for any after-hours activity, and this would be my last night here. Imagine what Mother would think of this!

At midnight, Costa turned the lights up and the music off, and paid me well for my shift. He was eager for me to continue to work for him. I was always up for an adventure wherever I went, but this was not a situation I needed to repeat for myself.

It was an awkward misunderstanding relayed through a friend of a friend of a friend. I had to laugh and see the funny side. Me! An escort in Greece – even if it was just for one night! I don't think I will be putting this on my resume!

Wink!

∼

Standing on the white, snowy slopes of Andorra, I dug my sticks firmly into the powdery ice and inched my way forward at a snail's pace. This skiing escapade had been high on my bucket list, and I couldn't believe I was here now, doing it for the first time.

I had picked up my skis, snowsuit, and accessories from the kiosk, and after a quick 10-minute tutorial – I was confident. It looked easy! I had ice skated as a teen and had great balance. How hard could it be? I pushed the points of my toes together in a V formation and shimmied forward in jerky movements. My loud, nervous squeals were embarrassing even for me. I mustered up all my courage and widened my style. Then – I was off! A little quicker than I anticipated. I went faster and faster down the mountain. I had no control of left or right. I just went full-steam ahead.

"Get out the way!" I shouted to unassuming competent skiers.

Their look of annoyance was evident. No one appreciates a novice skiing through the advanced zone. Apparently there are zones! And suddenly, I saw another girl screaming and out of control, heading straight for me.

We collided at full speed. Our arms, legs, skis, sticks, scarves, beanies, and dignity went every which way, and we ended up metres apart and flat on our backs. I thought *I'm going to die, right here, in Andorra on the snow!* I was winded and couldn't move.

The girl yelled out to me, "I'm so sorry, are you okay?" She was another novice tourist, and I suspected her skiing skills were on par with mine.

I shouted back honestly, "No, are you?" One of my legs was stinging from my ankle to my thigh.

She whimpered back – "I think I'm okay!" We shared a painful laugh. Before we could do anything else, two fit, handsome ski instructors had sliced up next to us. Speaking only in French, we weren't sure if they were talking to us or each other. As they helped us to our feet, it was apparent my leg was hurt quite badly.

I said to her, wincing through the pain, "Now you know my secret of how I attract European men!"

We laughed again. Laughing seemed to help with the acute humiliation and take my mind off the pain. The other girl seemed okay, and her instructor helped her back to the starting point of the run. I, on the other hand, had come off second best.

In very broken English, my instructor introduced himself as Valentin. He was strong, and did I mention he was handsome? Donned in a red and white tight-fitting, all-in-one snowsuit only made him even more captivating. With one swift movement, he hoisted me firmly into a piggyback grasp, pulled me onto his back, and proceeded down the ultrabright, white mountainous slope. I was nearly blinded. I had also lost my ski goggles.

He flew down at high speed, weaving left and right, and holding my thighs firmly while my arms were wrapped tightly around his neck in a koala embrace – the icy wind blowing against my squinted face. The tall, dark green pine trees positioned strategically in a row swished past us. I felt like I was in a movie. A James Bond movie – sexy, fast, and thrilling – although I'm sure for the locals looking on it was more like a scene from a Bridget Jones film!

Hurting my leg was worth it for *this* – a down the mountain ride on a hunky ski instructor's back. It was a once in a lifetime experience.

Valentin took me to the base of the mountain, where Dr Albert Einstein greeted me. Well, he looked very similar with little rimmed glasses and crazy white hair, and since nobody spoke any English, I had to formulate my own identities for everyone. But this man was the doctor for the ski lodge resort where I was staying. He tended to all the injured from the mountain, and I was his next casualty.

Trying to explain to a foreign doctor your invisible pain – who, by the way, can't speak any English – is a great challenge. He pushed and prodded, and I winced and cried. He scribbled on his chart accordingly, and then took some x-rays. After the doctor developed them, he explained them to me in French. Of course, I didn't understand a thing he said.

My leg was throbbing from my ankle to my groin. The doctor instructed me to lay straight on the metal bed. I had no idea what damage I had done. I couldn't make out anything he said to give me an idea of what was wrong with my leg. He put his hand on his heart, shook his head, and looked like he was going to cry.

Now I was getting scared. I needed to find someone from the hotel to interpret what the doctor was saying to me, but I couldn't walk. He started rattling around in the backroom, collecting instruments and clanging them into a large steel pan. He had bandages and tongs and lots of sharp metal things.

I started to panic; I tried to sit up. *OH, MY GOODNESS! HE IS GOING TO AMPUTATE MY LEG!* I wanted to show him my leg was feeling better and it wasn't so bad that – *HE HAD TO CUT IT OFF!* "*PLEASE NO!* I shouted, "*I DON'T WANT TO LOSE MY LEG!*"

I started to cry hysterically. The doctor heard me wailing and rushed over to show me the contents in his bucket. It was a thick white mixture. He made the motion of wiping it all over my leg. Now I understood. I was getting a plaster cast – not the removal of a limb! I relaxed back down and let him continue.

An hour later, I hobbled out of the medical cabin with a cast from ankle to thigh and very awkwardly caught the bus back to my hotel. A few hours later, and dosed up on painkillers, I sat by the fire in the front bar. I was a permanent fixture there for the rest of the week and became a bit of a tourist attraction. Word of my accident soon spread around the ski resort, and people from every different nationality came to the hotel just to sign my cast.

When I finally got back to London and went to the hospital, they discovered I had torn the cartilage in my knee. Of course, it healed, but very slowly – and I have never attempted the slopes again!

My travel adventures eventually came to an end. It was good to get back to Australia and all that was familiar. Although pleasantly distracted during my travels, the sting of my failed romance with Andrew was still excruciating.

At 25, my emotional internal wounds were crippling me. My dependency on alcohol increased, and I found myself drinking every day again to cope with life. I was an alcoholic, but I had no idea I was. My desperate quest for love was forever hopeful, so I straightened my happy mask of pretence, forced a smile, and took a shaky, drunk step of faith back into the dating world.

CHAPTER 11

Born to Charm

By the time I arrived back from my travels, my arms were considerably better for daily life. The Government office assessed my condition and diagnosed the tendons had still not repaired enough to resume typing. I was offered a clerical placement in another government department, which seemed perfect.

I was excited about a sea-change, and hopefully, this shift of tide would bring me something good. I didn't want much. Only one thing – that was, a good man to love, value, and protect me. That's all I ever wanted – all my life.

The sad thing was if good men crossed my path, like Bruce, I skilfully sabotaged these opportunities. My love radar was so damaged; my dating life was a dysfunctional mess.

The older I became, a pitiful panic seeped into my mind. I was terrified that no one would ever want me, and I would be alone forever.

I yearned for prince charming. My sub-conscience played havoc with my little girl dancing on the stage in front of the whole school. *Would my prince ever show up?* I knew he had to be out there somewhere. I craved to be loved so deeply; it was now an ugly obsession. Some might also call it – severe desperation.

I enjoyed my new job. It was very cruisy. No bosses to keep happy, and if we weren't busy, we were allowed to walk around the department and chat.

One day the lunch line in the canteen was busier than usual. As we casually shuffled along, I was having one of my regular, internal panic episodes, worrying if there was going to be a chicken and salad sandwich left by the time it was my turn. Lucky for me, there was, and I made my way back to the office block. My hands were full as I had grabbed an apple and a drink as well. I leaned against the heavy glass door, and in an awkward giraffe-like stance, tried to push it open with my back, when a hand reached out to help me. The door opened wide – *and there he stood!* Our eyes locked. A hot rush whooshed through my body. I felt myself blushing, and this made me blush even more.

"Thanks!" I said shyly.

"The pleasure is all mine," this gorgeous man replied with a grin, looking straight into me with his penetrating, pool-blue eyes. He emitted an aura that pulled me into him.

His large frame and wavy dark hair gave me goose-bumps, and instantly, I was captivated by his *charm*.

He purred, "You are new here, aren't you? I haven't seen your pretty face in the walkways of this block before." Riddled with panic, embarrassment, and a head full of nothing, I couldn't think of anything to say back to him, so I just giggled and smiled. As I walked away, I burned with humiliation and pondered how he must think I am the ditsiest brown-haired girl he has ever met.

For the rest of the afternoon, my questions plagued me. *Who was this man? What was his name? Was he single?* I prayed to God for us to meet again. I have to confess – I didn't pray to God anymore – only when I wanted things, and every time I did, I felt a little bit guilty. But I *really* wanted to go out with this guy because his eyes were just so blue, and his voice was just so, aaahhhhh, *dreamy*.

Then it started; the taunts of my inner rival! *He's never going to like you! There is NO way he will be attracted to you! He most definitely thinks you are fat and ugly!* On cue, my resident monster blew his whistle to umpire the game of; *Emma's insecurities and self-hate* versus *a wishful reality*. With great enthusiasm, they ran out into the field of my mind to play.

Keeping the score of my two opponents was tormenting. On one side – obsessive, hopeful prayer – fought with – compulsive, destructive, internal dialogue. They took turns to speak over and over inside my head. I was used to living this way, but it was always exhausting. I tried very hard to relax and sit on the sidelines and shut off from my prayerful begging and self-ridicule. I always lost.

Over the next few weeks, I couldn't see him anywhere at work. Where was he? I drove myself insane with desperation. I prayed every night to God pleading we would cross paths again. And we did; at a nightclub in Perth. He was standing at the bar, and without knowing it was him, I politely asked if I could move through to the counter to order a drink. To our surprise, here we were again – locking eyes. Was this a divine appointment? It felt like one. I thanked God under my breath for giving me what I fiercely wanted.

His name was Alan Janse. He bought me a drink, and we chatted for hours. And he arranged a future date with me. He did like me, AND he wanted me to be his girlfriend! Woohoo! Internal happy dance! After being emotionally ravaged by Andrew, maybe life was going to be fantastic for me, after all?

In the weeks that followed, we became inseparable. I stayed over at Alan's house most nights, and we just – *chilled*. He wasn't a big talker, so we didn't share much in the way of conversation, but at least I was not alone. My parents were very wary of him, but nothing they said would deter me from being by his side.

Alan gripped my fragile tapestry firmly in his hands. He embroidered his fancy new threads with such precision. They were detailed, intricate, and a very dark shade; woven with great skill.

Our relationship was a decadent, chaotic whirlwind. We drank ridiculous amounts of alcohol together, either at home or at the pub. I soon discovered he smoked a lot of marijuana, or pot, as we called it in the '80s. I didn't want to smoke anymore – but I did. I wasn't going to do anything to jeopardise this relationship.

We would drink, get stoned, then take speed and go with the flow of where the night's stream would take us. Of course, the drugs took us both to vile places, and in our heightened state of euphoria were both unfaithful to each other at the decadent parties we attended.

We thought we were having fun at these wild fiestas – but because of the drugs, our behaviour became selfishly unshackled, which always ended up in wild debauchery. We weren't rock stars, but we led a lifestyle of sex, drugs, and rock and roll. Alan's crowd was as untamed as he was, and every time we mixed drugs and alcohol, there were no restraints on our ego's appetite.

There was no deep love between Alan and me and being unfaithful to each other was not the relationship I wanted. Behaving so loosely in my morals was *not who I was*. But I was a slave to my addictions; the drug-master was in charge, and I was trapped. My morals and ethics were compromised, and I was compelled by a dark inner force to do things I didn't want to do. I was on a fast, downhill track, and I couldn't get off. But part of me didn't care about that anyway. Alan said he loved me, he wanted to be with me, and that was all that mattered.

But it wasn't long before Alan and I started having fights over lies he had told me. Money was going missing from my purse. Strange girls were phoning him. He had a quick answer for everything, usually resulting in me always having to say I'm sorry. I couldn't see beneath his bewitching personality; he was a skilled pathological liar and a narcissist. My empathetic nature, low self-esteem, and acute anxiety made me easy prey for his demise. They say love is blind, *and I was*. I couldn't see we were highly toxic together. We were not a match made in heaven. We were a match made in hell. But the thought of me being single wasn't an option, so I persevered in the hope that I could change him and things would get better.

When Alan asked me to marry him – everything inside me screamed – *NO, DON'T DO IT!* I knew in my gut; I couldn't trust his shallow character – but my insecurities were more significant than my common sense.

I justified my panic. We had fun, even if it was only because we smoked pot together. Surely all of Alan's dysfunction – which I was sure

I could fix – was going to be better than being alone and unloved. *Something* was better than nothing. Right?

Yes – this was a terrible foundation to build a relationship on – but sad to say – it was mine. I was 26 and unmarried. In the '80s, any age past 25, you were considered a spinster. All of my friends were married and having babies. Petrified of being *left on the shelf* and completely missing the love boat, I wasn't going to let this proposal pass by me.

I gave Alan my answer. I said – *Yes* – and the wedding plans began. I wanted to get married using my Grandma's wedding ring, but Alan was against that idea and firmly said NO! My childhood dream to wear my Grandma's ring would never be. I was desperate to please him. I didn't want to do anything to stop him from marrying me. So, Alan soon became the dictator in our relationship – and I let him. My internal screams were loud – *Don't marry him!* But I convinced myself it was just cold feet.

Our wedding day soon arrived. It was late October, and we had hoped for lovely weather. Not too hot and not too cold. Growing up in a Methodist home, Mother and Dad persuaded us to have a Christian ceremony. Alan and I were so far away from anything that resembled a Christian lifestyle, but deep down, I wanted God to bless our marriage. I needed all the help I could get.

Our traditional stone church was beautiful. It had stained glass windows and detailed hand-carved wooden pews. An array of fresh flowers added to the finishing touch of elegance. Vibrant colours of red, gold, and purple – spoke of royalty – fit for a king and queen. It was the perfect setting for a fairy tale wedding. That was where the perfection stopped.

The day was a disaster. It began with the flowers in the bridesmaid's bouquets being the wrong colour, and they clashed terribly with everything else. The limousine was extremely late to pick me up, and we couldn't contact them. Everyone suspected they had forgotten the booking. Standing around, waiting in the driveway at home gave me an anxiety episode. Then the weather turned cold. It became gloomy with dark clouds casting a grey misery over the day. Of course, it rained, and my delicately curled hair volumised to an unflattering frizz. The organist for the church didn't turn up. One of my mother's friends could play the organ, so she jumped up promptly and played any tune to save the moment.

Dad walked me down a long aisle, which felt more like a slow, funeral march than a joyous occasion. Alan stood waiting for me at the front of the church, swaying strangely. He didn't look well. I soon discovered his condition was self-inflicted. Spiced with pot and alcohol, Alan slurred his vows. His chuckles were very inappropriate in the silent pin-drop moments. I was furious. Alan told me many times marijuana was his number one priority in his life. This day confirmed it. I should have done a 'runaway bride' but I just couldn't. As the Minister recited our vows: for better or for worse; in sickness and in health; till death do us part, I reluctantly said – *I do* – and became Mrs Emma Janse.

We were expecting our first child. Knowing I could finally share an identity with another human being in this world made me incredibly happy. I can't explain the feeling of love I had for this tiny human being growing inside me. This baby was my heart, my joy, my life. I was going to be the best mother I could. No matter what sacrifice I had to make, my unborn child came first.

I gave up drugs and alcohol immediately. It was easy for me to stop our party lifestyle when I became pregnant. I had internal responsibilities, but Alan didn't have to – and didn't. He got stoned most days and drunk every night. Very quickly, we grew apart. Now, I was married to a complete stranger, with nothing in common.

Alan was often home late from work, working double shifts, or not coming home at all. He was terrible at managing our finances. Money went missing from our bank account, and overdue bills were piling high. A few times, he said he lost his pay packet. Who does that?

Our baby boy was born, and we called him Nathan. It means a gift of God. In the middle of my turmoil, living with Alan's dysfunction, Nathan indeed was a gift to my life. Nathan gave me a purpose for living, and he was the joy in my day. Alan was jealous of Nathan. My sole attention was not on Alan, and this made him angry. He dove deeper into his confessed first love, marijuana. The distance between us intensified.

Because my parents were financially comfortable – coupled with generous hearts – for our wedding gift they bought us: a block of land; a newly-built house; $20,000 for furnishings; a landscaped garden; and a car. They wanted us to have a good start in life, but this made Alan angry. He was outraged that my parents were interfering in our lives. Funnily enough, he received the charity happily with open arms while cursing my parents behind their backs.

Alan took charge of all our finances, and I had no say. Despite every dollar my parents gave us, we never had enough. They continued to pay our overdue bills and bought our food. They couldn't bear to see our newborn baby and me going without daily necessities: electricity, water, bread, and milk. In our first year of marriage, their cheque butts totalled $100,000. They frequently lectured me about managing our money. Of course, I felt guilty, but I had no control over anything. Alan was our frivolous financial planner. I never knew where any of the money was going. He could have had a secret bank account for all I knew. There was nothing I could do. Alan lived in a state of continual disarray – in *every* area of his life.

Trapped in this unfortunate marriage dynamic, the only thing that eased my pain was denial; denial of Alan's never-ending lies and selfish behaviour, his control and manipulation and lack of provision for his family, and his continual put-downs. But brushing off his actions didn't stop reality. Alan wore me down so much I had no voice in our marriage. He blocked me from seeing my friends. His reasons against other people were always justified. If he couldn't find fault with them just the fact that he didn't like them severed any further contact.

I became Alan's puppet, and he pulled my strings. It wasn't long before he controlled my every move. In my mind, I wanted to escape, but I couldn't leave. I had a child to think of, and my wedding vows rang loudly in my ears. *For better or for worse, in sickness and in health, till death do us part.*

I wasn't an actively religious person, but we had been married in the sight of God. To me, that was a serious commitment, and one which I couldn't be flippant with just because things might be getting hard. I knew most marriages went through their rough patches at times, and I was faithfully going to endure our tough seasons and do all I could to honour my vows.

But if there was such a thing as – *a life of hell on earth* – I was living it.

The last time I prayed to God, I was desperate to be with Alan. Now, I was frantic with a new prayer. *Please, God, make Alan stop controlling and dominating me.* I felt guilty for only talking to God when I wanted something, but daily life with Alan was becoming unbearable, and each day I was more desperate.

Do you believe God answers prayers? I do. But not always in the way we imagine. And our answered prayers can come in a way, and at a time, we least expect it. Mine did.

One day Alan's lying mouth tripped him up. He was spinning his usual tales about where our money had gone. The more he talked, the less sense he made. Eventually, he spiralled down into a hole, and he couldn't claw his way back out.

The elephant in the room was visible to both of us. Two years of enduring a terrible marriage, I couldn't live like this anymore. Our relationship was utterly hopeless. I was worn down and exhausted. With tears in my eyes, I pleaded desperately, "Alan, what sort of marriage do we have if you keep lying to me about – *everything?*"

I expected a fight, and to be silenced and suppressed. I expected Alan to flip into one of his rages and punch the wall. He did this when things weren't going his way. I expected him to dominate and intimidate me with his fierce glare. But nothing prepared me for what he did next.

Alan hung his head and said nothing. He walked into the bedroom, packed an overnight bag, shuffled past me and walked out the door as if I was invisible. That was it – no goodbyes to his one-year-old son or me. Alan just left. I had no idea where he was going. Alan never phoned. No one else knew where he had gone either. He just vanished from our lives.

Little did I know, a bit further up ahead, *something greater* was waiting for me.

CHAPTER 12

Divine Appointment

Alan had now been gone six months, still with no contact. I saw his desertion as a brand-new start, but I felt incredibly lost. Yearning to be loved more than ever before, I went out on a few dates, but none were successful. Fresh layers of rejection coated the rejection I already had. I was in a terrible state.

Desperate to find some lovely friends, the only caring and decent people I remembered having in my life were the girls and guys at the youth group. Everyone was kind and full of deep inner happiness, and they genuinely cared for one another. That's what I wanted.

I began to pray for God to help me. Yes, I only prayed to God when I wanted things, but something was changing in my heart this time when I prayed – I felt a genuine reverent surrender.

My darling mother's words resounded in my head. *When one door closes, another one will open.* Just that one little phrase, at this time in my life, gave me the hope to press on.

I found a job working part-time selling make-up in a large department store. Veronica, a vibrant, sassy red-head, worked the same shift as me. Instantly, we clicked. We chattered behind our counters when we weren't busy. Ronnie, as we called her, had two small children and had also broken up with her partner. We shared our sorrows and cheered one another up as best we could.

Ronnie came into work one day, and she was *shining*. Her radiant countenance was so visible; I was busting to ask her what had happened. Maybe she had found a new boyfriend? Her answer was not what I expected. Ronnie's cousin, who was a Christian, had given Ronnie a Bible for her birthday, and she had been reading it.

Keeping a low voice, Ronnie whispered, "Please don't laugh at me Em when I tell you, I have started praying, and it feels wonderful!" She didn't want any of the other staff members to hear her and think she was turning into a religious freak.

I whispered back, "Oh… Ronnie, of course, I won't laugh at you! I think that's great if it makes you feel good. Now I am going to tell *you* something. Don't you laugh at me either, I have started praying to God too, AND… *I even gave my heart to Jesus when I was 14 on a youth camp!*"

I hoped that made her feel a little more at ease – though funnily enough when I said it, part of me felt proud – in an awkward kind of way.

She continued whispering, "I've been reading the Psalms, and feeling happier and peaceful inside, especially about the kids' loser dad."

I cheered her on, "Ronnie, go for it! Whatever makes you happy! I honestly don't think you are a nut!"

We had a little giggle together and a reassuring hug. As we embraced something invisible grabbed hold of me. A pressure. A presence. It wouldn't go away. I had no idea what it was. It was as though a rope had lassoed firmly around my heart and started pulling me towards God.

This presence got stronger every day, and now it consumed my heart, my mind, and my body.

After a week of this intense pressure and presence, I had to address it. I phoned Ronnie and shared this remarkable phenomenon to see if she knew what was happening.

"Emma, you're just becoming aware of God around you. Can you hang on a sec? I'll grab my Bible. I want to read to you something I read today."

As I waited for her to come back, the essence around me became heavier.

"Em, are you there?" I was – only just! Ronnie continued, "Listen to this, 'Matthew 7 verse 13 and 14, Jesus says, enter by the narrow gate. For wide is the gate and broad is the way that leads to destruction, and there are many who go in by it. Because narrow is the gate and difficult is the way which leads to life, and there are few who find it.' See Em, God says, without Him the majority of people in the world are on the broad road to destruction, but the way of Jesus is narrow and not many find it. Can't you see that's exactly how we live in the world today?"

I started feeling lightheaded, and I knew I had to lie down. "Wow, that is incredible! Thanks, Ronnie, I have to go now, though. I will talk to you later."

I went into my bedroom and lay down on the bed. I hoped as I rested the presence would ease off. I started to think about what Ronnie had read and what it meant. I closed my eyes and instantly I saw a road in front of me. This vision was tangible, as though I had transported to another dimension.

It was an *enormous*, wide road, not made from tar, but from steel – silvery in appearance – and when you looked down, it was so shiny you could see your reflection – just like a mirror. It was hard and cold. No warmth radiated from this road. I sensed it calling me to walk on it, so I decided I would see where it went.

Immediately, as my foot touched the metal, a feeling of insecurity penetrated right through to the core of my being, and I felt incredibly lonely. I saw a large gathering of people in the distance, and I heard the faint sound of wild celebration. Out of my human need for love, I eagerly ventured forward. With each step forward, the noise ahead became louder. Music thumped amidst chatter and laughter, and the atmosphere was raging. I started to feel excited.

I couldn't wait to go and join the party.

As I walked along this vast road, I casually glanced over to my left. I saw ten brown, wooden sign-posts. They were erected just past the edge of this road. Relatively small in height, you wouldn't notice them unless you looked purposefully. Each had an inscription, but I couldn't make out what they said, so out of curiosity, I made my way over to have a closer look. The words on the signs were definite warnings of what was ahead on this broad, shiny path. I could tell they had been written by hand and burnt into the wood.

DANGER. DEATH. DESTRUCTION. DISASTER. DISEASE. DOWNFALL. DEVASTATION. DISILLUSIONMENT. DESPAIR.

The last sign-post was blank.

I was very apprehensive now about proceeding, and as I stood there cautiously, I could feel something else starting to radiate from within the wood itself, and a beautiful serenity settled around me. As I tuned into this beautiful essence, words appeared on the last signpost.

DON'T GO AHEAD! The air around me became pure love.

As I looked past the wooden signs, I noticed a little red dusty track with a thick cloud of peace hovering over it. You couldn't see this small track from the vast road. It only became apparent when you took the time to stop and look. There was no music, nor people, although loneliness was not evident.

Then I saw Him! *Jesus!* He suddenly appeared on the little red dusty track. His eyes were full of love and compassion for *me!* Jesus was beautiful in every way. He was pure, and I wanted to fall to my knees and cry. I never in my whole life felt a love so deep and all-consuming. Jesus reached out His hands beckoning me to come into His arms and surrender my entire life so He could love me forever.

Suddenly, I became distracted by the noises ahead on the shiny, hard road. They became increasingly louder. Volumes of shrieking and laughter erupted in the distance. Thoughts rushed through my mind – *I'm missing out on something that's happening up there*. The noise itself started to pull me away from Jesus, and it took all my human effort to try and focus on His love for me. I felt torn and confused. Do I stay here or go and check out what appears to be an electrifying good time? I hesitated.

I believed in God, but I didn't want to get involved with religion. But the love from Jesus was so overwhelmingly beautiful; I didn't want to leave. I didn't feel pressured by Jesus. It was my choice if I wanted to stay, so I thought I would.

As I made that decision in my heart, a shadowy voice of a supernatural entity, similar, although far higher than a human, powerfully expressed words that absorbed into my whole being. Flashes, like lightning bolts, went through me. These tangible natural elements must be God, I thought. I felt porous to this supreme power. The divine voice boomed like thunder all around me.

"LIFE…"

A breath of wind brushed my hair softly across my face as it filled me with passion and purpose.

"LOVE…"

I tingled as a red mist of pure adoration settled around me.

I stood still in total awe, receiving a saturation of whatever the voice had spoken.

"LAUGHTER…"

Giggles welled up inside me, and I was full of joy.

"LASTING…"

I closed my eyes and inhaled pure air that would endure for all eternity.

"LUSTRE…"

Everything glorious and beautiful was mine if I chose this narrow dusty path.

"LONGING…"

A significant drop of shimmering hope fell from above, as if in slow motion. I reached out, caught it, and held it carefully, trying not to let it roll from the palm of my hand. I instinctively knew God would give me more drops. I simply had to ask.

"COME…"

The last word scared me.

Immediately, I knee-jerked back to my reality of who I was. My head spun. Fear gripped me, and I broke out in a cold sweat. I began to panic, and my heart started thumping. I felt dirty and unclean, unworthy of receiving anything so beautiful. All my insecurities ignited within me and pushed away any love and life offered by God and mine to have. Instantly, I became aware that I was standing on the cold, steel path once again.

I looked down at my reflection. *I was so ugly*. Thoughts of self-hate sped around in my head at a fast rate, saying over and over; *you are worthless and deserve nothing! Only people of value are allowed on the red, dusty path and – YOU ARE A NOBODY! How could you ever think that God would want YOU?*

But the love I felt was SO genuine. I was confused. The red path or the steel road? I tried to get clarity by reasoning the whole thing through in my mind. I wanted to be with people, and I needed a touch of physical affection, not just vapours, and mists. I believed in Jesus, but the invitation He offered me required my whole life. What does that even mean? If I press on ahead on the steel road, the road I am comfortable and familiar with, I might find my purpose in this life. Plus, how did I know this wasn't a trap on the dusty path? I couldn't see where it was going to lead me. It was scary to take a giant leap of faith into the unknown.

The crowd in the distance became even louder, and I made my final decision. I'm going to go to the party! Instantly, the life-giving essence vanished, and I became aware that now, I was totally on my own. I turned and ran toward the multitudes. I wondered if they had all passed this supernatural being as well and had to choose like I did. I ran as fast as I could on the cold road of steel.

I suddenly smelt a repulsive odour. It was similar to the foul stench of a stagnant pond. It soon eased off, or I became used to it – one of the two – because, after a while, it didn't bother me. There were millions of people. Young, old, rich, poor, black, white, famous, and not. It was very noisy. It was impossible to hear what anyone was saying to each other. With the constant loud music playing, everyone had to shout.

It sure was one big, extravagant rave party. The laser lights, smoke machines, and fireworks created an exciting atmosphere. I wanted to make friends, but no one noticed or spoke to me. Everyone was so wrapped up in their own life, doing their own thing, I made no impression on them at all.

A group of well-groomed men and women were looking down, admiring themselves in the mirrored surface. Their smiles were false, as they pretended nothing else mattered, so long as they were satisfied with how they looked. Absorbed by their self-image, they had no time for each other, let alone me.

I thought it might get friendlier as I travelled further along the shiny, wide road, so I pressed on. Some people were dancing. I love dancing, so I joined in. But again, I was ignored. Others were stumbling drunk, popping pills, and injecting needles. In the middle of this chaos, couples were having sex in front of everyone without embarrassment or shame. And others had formed group orgies. Nothing was sacred or pure.

I heard gunshots in the distance, and I was frightened. I didn't want to advance, but I couldn't stay in this toxic atmosphere. I found it extremely hard to take in everything that was happening. As I moved on, I saw another group of people. They were fighting and killing each other, and wars were raging in full force. Hate filtered through the air, and death hovered in delight. Everything was out of control.

The saddest thing I saw was the innocent children influenced by this evil display. They had no choice but to copy the same behaviour and lifestyle of everything they saw.

There was also another realm on this road. Out of the dark shadows, demonic beings subtly appeared and mingled between everyone giving more alcohol, drugs, and weapons to whoever they could. Whatever people wanted; those fiends of darkness made it available. But they were just the messengers.

Ruling over this road was a creature – otherwise known as – *Prince of the Air*. It was the most demonic, vicious, evil, wicked supernatural being in the world. This monster was a combination of a reptile and a human being. It wasn't big and didn't stand out, but its supreme power and authority seduced everyone into submission and falsehood.

Its eyes burned like red fire and penetrated right through you. Its horny head could rotate entirely in a circle, so it knew what was happening with everyone, at any time. Flicking out a black tongue covered in razor-sharp spikes, it could cut you into tiny pieces with one lash. If you didn't bow down to its authority and kingship, a sacrifice of flesh was taken by force from you or your household. The creature's only delight was to rob, kill, and destroy. Its depraved agenda fed its sick desires and gave it a sense of grandeur and importance.

The accumulated debauchery from everyone on this road ascended as sweet, smelling worship, inhaled through its nostrils. It paraded around like a powerful parasite, feeding on the flesh of its helpless and unaware victims. Deceiving and devouring humanity is how it sustained its spiritual strength.

It hated God, and the two kingdoms of good and evil were in a constant battle against each other. It knew God was incredibly more beautiful, powerful, and majestic, so it kept every person as far away as possible from hearing how much God loved them.

Although I didn't want to go any further, I knew I had to see everything on this path. I pressed past the wars and bloodshed, and up ahead, I saw a low, black cloud. Black particles of air sprinkled down like pepper from the dark condensed mist. These particles were diseases and viruses that were very much alive and programmed with assignments of death.

A wind carried the deadly germs far and wide and landed on many innocent bystanders.

I heard more people wailing and screaming in pain and torture. Some had visible physical injuries from the wars, drug abuse, and violence, but some didn't appear damaged in any way. They looked quite normal and healthy. Men, women, and children. I got closer to see if I could work out what their distress was.

There was one attractive lady who was grasping her head. She was hyperventilating and convulsing with fear. Gripped with intense pain, she couldn't stop the voices, the stabbing sensations in her mind. As I looked around, there were so many people with the same illness. I could feel the torment in each one. Then it dawned on me. I knew why these people were suffering. It was because of all the illnesses you can't see and the many insipid, depressive, mental-health conditions. These people were just like me – this road was the saddest thing I had ever seen.

I looked down, overwhelmed with grief, and saw my reflection again. Suddenly, I was held captive by my own tormented life. I couldn't bear standing on this broad, shiny, metal road any longer. I had to get off it. I wanted to go back to the beginning of this journey. I had to find the red, dusty track again, where the supreme, supernatural essence tried to surround me with love and laughter and all good things. How could I get back there? Could I even get back there? Why on earth was I seeing all this? I couldn't stay on this road a second longer.

I sat up. I was incredibly hot. I went into the bathroom to splash cold water on my face. I looked flushed. Staring at my reflection in the mirror, I started crying, and I had no idea why. I couldn't stop. I stood there in the bathroom and sobbed. *I will never forget in my whole life what happened next.*

The supernatural presence I had just felt on the red, dusty path, encapsulated me inside a bubble. It was so strong and intense; I found it hard to breathe. The spiritual presence was not easing off. Instead, it was getting more intense, so I decided to talk to it.

"Okay, you have been following me for the past week. I'm not sure why and I don't know what you want with me, but okay, you have my attention. I think what I'm feeling is you, God! I've been praying to you, and you know my life is a mess, and I need help, but what's happening to me now? *What is all THIS?*"

There was no response from this spiritual essence.

I asked again, "I feel you want something from me, but I don't know what it is? *GOD, WHAT DO YOU WANT FROM ME?*"

I saw a portal to heaven open up above me in my bathroom, and I felt God himself looking down on me. I wasn't scared. I felt peaceful. All of a sudden, I realised, this spiritual sensation had appeared to me once before in my life. It was at the youth camp when Jesus had come to me at the end of my bed. Now I had just felt it again on the red, dusty path.

Another wave of presence flowed over me. Instantly I was overwhelmed with the reality of people in my life not wanting me. My birth mother and father. Graham. Jake and Andrew. Past friends. And now, Alan.

Now I knew what God wanted! He wanted to talk to me about *this!* I broke down and sobbed from the depth of my soul.

"Why, God? Why do people not want me? Why do people in my life – ALWAYS LEAVE ME?"

Still, there was no response. I looked up through the portal to heaven. Every part of me was crumbling.

"WHY, GOD? WHY DOES EVERYONE LEAVE ME?"

Immediately, I felt another spiritual presence appear in the corner of the bathroom. With every heightened sense in my being, and clarity of mind, *I knew it was JESUS!* I couldn't see Him as a person like I did at the youth camp that night, but the essence of His presence and His voice was the same as He spoke gently, *"Remember what I said to you – I WILL NEVER LEAVE YOU, I WILL NEVER FORSAKE YOU."*

Waves of love and acceptance flowed over me. *Of course, I remembered! How could I forget?* Then a voice boomed audibly through the open ceiling. I knew this was God.

"YOU GAVE YOUR HEART, BUT YOU DIDN'T GIVE YOUR LIFE. I WANT YOUR HEART AND YOUR LIFE!"

Now I was scared. What on earth was going on? The essence, the presence, the voice, I had no explanation for it.

I mustered up some courage. "Okay," I spoke out loud.

"If this is *You*, God, asking me to become a Christian, I don't think I'll make a good one! I've done drugs, and I drink. I've slept around in my past. I never go to church. I'm just not cut out to be a goodie-goodie church person!"

There was no reply. None of that seemed to bother God, and the presence just got heavier. I felt there was no escape, and I didn't know what to do. I had to think quickly! So, I came up with a plan. A proposition to present to God because – honestly – that's the only thing I came up with on the spot.

I spoke with real intention.

"Let's try this, God. Here is my hand," I said, holding up my right arm towards the ceiling.

"Let's hold hands for three days, and then at the end of that, we can decide. I mean, you might think I won't make a good Christian, and I might not want to become one either. Fair deal?"

I felt God take hold of my right hand and beginning at my feet; a white, all-consuming fire began to burn slowly up inside my whole body. Porous to this supreme substance, I couldn't move. I stood as still as a statue. Riveted in front of the mirror with my eyes wide open, I witnessed what took place next. In a flash, a black veil that had been covering my eyes all my life whisked off my face. I saw it go.

Instantly, incredible joy came upon me and filled me, and I overflowed with giggles. I had never known happiness like this ever before in my life. Pure love, as white as snow sprinkled down all around me. It melted and washed away every bad thing in my life. Large drops of hope like a gentle rain fell as floating bubbles bursting upon my life as they touched my skin.

I was receiving all the pure essences God had offered me on the red, dusty path.

I felt Jesus pouring His love into me, giving me peace and excitement for life. I felt as though I had just won lotto – ten times over! *I wanted to burst – I felt so happy.* I looked at myself in the mirror. I was different. My brown eyes were full of light; my face was shining, just like Ronnie's face had shined. I *felt* different. I couldn't explain it. Maybe no one would believe me, but it had happened. It happened to me. *I had just had an encounter with God.*

I had to find a Bible. I knew I had one stashed in a box in the shed from high school. I found it and opened it up at random. My fingers ran across the page as I read. "Joshua 1 verse 5 – Jesus says, I will not leave you; I will not forsake you." WOW! That is in the Bible. I never knew that! It was crazy! I closed it and opened it again. "John 14 verse 27 – Jesus says, Peace I leave with you. My peace I give to you, not as the world gives, do I give to you." AMAZING! Because I could feel peace!

Then it dawned on me! Of course, the cold, hard, steel road was the world we live in today! I had lived on this road with my drug and alcohol addiction, my self-loathing, and my Godless lifestyle. Revelation upon revelation poured into me like a computer updating with the latest software. Old files of prior knowledge and understanding now were being replaced with new downloads of spiritual reality and truth.

I saw the devil in the world for who he was, and even though he is not visible, I knew it doesn't mean he doesn't exist! I saw so clearly that the world is suffering because these two kingdoms of light and darkness are always in total opposition with each other. God loves everyone in the world and wants a relationship with each one, and Satan hates God and will do everything in his power to stop that happening. God is pure love, and the devil is pure hate. God is healing, and the devil is destruction in every way possible. I saw how the devil had been trying to destroy my life, but today – God showed up and intervened.

Overwhelmed, I went to lie down again. I closed my eyes to focus on God. I thanked Him for showing Himself to me in such a real way. I thanked Him because even though people had left me in my life – Jesus *never* did.

I saw another vision of a staircase. I assumed it led to heaven, so I started to climb it. With each step, my body changed, and by the time I reached the top, I had gone from an adult, back to being a little girl.

As I stood at the top of the stairs, I saw Him. Yes! I saw God. He had white hair and an even whiter long beard and an incredibly kind face. He wore a pure white robe, but it wasn't about what He wore – instead – it was all about – WHO HE WAS.

An essence of love poured out from Him, like tumultuous waves crashing on the shore. They never stopped. Wave after wave, God's love kept pouring into me, drenching me. I was completely saturated! It's incredibly hard to put into words, but God's love was so fierce and pure, it shone brighter than the sun. He was every element of nature, and He was more powerful than anything in this world and universe.

God sat in an elaborate, gold chair covered in jewels. It was breathtaking. He waved to me like Father Christmas does when it is your turn to sit on his knee after a long wait. Except there was no wait. There was no one else here but *me*. God was all mine, and I was all His. I climbed up and sat on His lap. His arms wrapped around me, keeping me safe, secure, and protected.

God was my Father, my Daddy, my Papa, and I was His precious daughter. He was so proud and adored me – for just being me. I felt it. I knew it.

There was something God had wanted me to know my whole life, but I had never allowed Him ever to get close enough to tell me. As I sat on God's knee, He looked deep into my eyes and said, "Emma, I love you. I have always loved you, and I will always love you, for you are, and always will be, my child."

CHAPTER 13

A Brand New Life

I was now *a born-again Christian!* I always thought born-again Christians had lost the plot. It was acceptable to call yourself a Christian, but a born-again Christian – now you are just weird! Except I didn't feel weird at all. I felt amazing! I felt so clean and fresh on the inside. My old, dirty, stained sinful life had been washed by God's purifying, forgiving love, and my spirit was bursting with hope. I had been born once from my mother's womb, and now, born again by God's Spirit. It was unbelievable to my natural mind, but after my spiritual awakening, it was clear.

Through my encounter, God gave me new eyes to look through. The grass was greener. The sky was bluer. The flowers danced with abundant life. Somehow, when the black veil whisked off my eyes, everything became more precise and brighter to my spiritual and natural senses. The world hadn't changed dramatically – I had.

Peace resided in and around me continuously. This peace calmed my mind, relaxed my body, and energised my heart. I was spiritually alive!

The negative, dark voices I had lived with all my life were gone. Jesus came to set me free. I was free, indeed!

Now my tapestry was being woven with God's pure, gold threads of love that were changing the very fabric of my being. I would sit and read my Bible for hours. I would pray and talk to God like He was an old friend sitting right next to me. *I never felt alone.* If this was to be my life now on the red, dusty path, it was incredible!

I had this opportunity before to walk this path at 14 when I found Jesus at the youth camp, but I had walked away from Him. This time, nothing was going to distract me from following Jesus.

I prayed, "God lead me to a church, one that is perfect for Nathan and me." A few days later, I crossed paths with Jessie, my old friend. I hadn't seen her in years. Last time I saw her we were running scared and thankful to be alive. Jessie shared that she had become a Christian. Seeing Jessie was not a coincidence! I shared my bathroom encounter, and she listened with excitement. I told her I was looking for a church and of course, she invited me to hers. It was called New Beginning Ministries. Although it was a 40-minute drive from my house, I knew this church was the one. Sunday came, and Nathan and I, dressed in our best, set off on our new adventure.

I was nervous as I entered the foyer. People were friendly and welcoming. There was a buzz of excitement. Nathan couldn't wait to jump out of my arms and play with the other children in Sunday School.

I walked down a very long corridor to the main auditorium. It was modern and colourful with banners and flags strung around the walls and ceiling. There was a warm hum in the atmosphere as people greeted each other, some shaking hands and others hugging, but all happy to be in church. Suddenly, a scream pierced the air. I looked over to see who made such a squeal. It was – *Leanne!* Yes, from the youth camp. She ran over and threw her arms around me. We were both shocked to see each other.

"Oh Emma," Leanne exclaimed excitedly, "I haven't stopped praying for you. I heard you went into the drug scene, and I was so worried about you. Praise Jesus; He has brought you back. It's so wonderful to see you!"

Her remark floored me. I hadn't seen her for over ten years, and to think she still thought of me, let alone prayed for me, really touched me. Her genuine heart that I knew back then shone through again. If anything, she looked more radiant. We caught up on the years passed, and she was sorry to hear Alan had walked out. She was happily married to a beautiful Christian man, with baby number three on the way. The Pastor of this church was a young man named *Frank*. Yes, that's right! The Youth Pastor at the Easter camp that year. The youth group had grown into a church. I couldn't believe it. Another coincidence? I don't think so! It was obvious God had led me back to the same path I had travelled once before. It felt so comfortable here, just like home.

We sang modern songs and old hymns, and at times it felt like I touched heaven, mainly when they played Amazing Grace: *I once was lost, but now I'm found, Was blind, but now I see*. I wondered if the person who wrote this song had a bathroom experience like mine.

There was an altar call at the end of the service for people who wanted prayer. I don't remember walking forward, but I found myself standing at the front of the church. The songs seemed to get louder as waves of God's presence crashed over me, and I couldn't stop my tears flowing.

A lady came up behind me, placed her hand on my back, and started praying. She spoke to me quietly. "Have you ever been to Paris?" I had travelled there on Gordon. I nodded, and she continued praying. Then she spoke again but this time very quietly. "I see something, but I don't want to say what I see because I don't want to upset you."

As the tears rolled down my cheeks, I gave her permission to tell me. She moved closer to me and whispered. "I see a terminated baby, and it is trying to climb up the side of a grey metal bucket… and I keep getting the word, Paris? I'm not quite sure how the two are connected? Do you know what this means?"

I knew what this meant – my abortion. I crumbled to the ground sobbing. I couldn't stop myself and groaned with deep pain. Not a physical pain; a spiritual pain. A spiritual force of grief, shame, anger and regret.

I fought off my emotions to calm down and gathered my strength and whispered, "Yes, I know what this means. I had an abortion, and I named my baby Paris! I didn't want to have an abortion, I know

I killed my baby, I know it was wrong. I'm so sorry; I'm so sorry!" The release of this trapped secret erupted another wave of flowing tears.

Gently, the lady spoke softly, "Come to the Pastor's office; we can pray privately there." The presence of God was so heavily upon me; I needed help to walk to the room. She sat me down in a comfortable chair.

"My name is Rose, and I am an intercessor in this church. If you are happy to do so, I will lead you in a prayer to forgive yourself and to ask God for His forgiveness."

"Yes, Rose, please," I answered, "I want you to." As I repeated the prayer for God to forgive me and another prayer for me to forgive myself, waves of love and healing pulsated through me, washing me clean on the inside from all my disdain.

Rose explained, "The precious blood of Jesus shed for you on the cross wipes away all your sins, and God has forgiven you."

I replied, "Thank you, Rose, for praying with me." I felt forgiven by God. I felt His overwhelming love and grace.

Rose spoke gently again, "You will see your baby one day in heaven."

I asked her, "How do you know that?"

Rose answered, "We believe aborted babies go straight to heaven as they are never born into sin. God's ways are greater than our ways."

I sat fully enveloped in a substantial peace. I felt like I was drunk, and I was, but not with alcohol. A pure essence of the Holy Spirit had inebriated me. "God loves you very much," Rose said. "God knows you right to the very core of your being, and He wants the very best for you. Jesus will always be there to help. Never forget that. It doesn't matter what you have done or will ever do; God will always forgive you and never reject you. Always come to Him with everything, even if you think it is such a small thing, it doesn't matter, God cares." After what had just happened to me, I had to agree.

No one knew I called my aborted baby, Paris. I never told anyone. But God knew, and He loved me enough to take away all my guilt and shame. God forgave me and let me know through this beautiful lady.

We had a hug, and I sat quietly for a little while before I had to collect Nathan. Coming to church was *nothing* like I thought it was going to be. It was a place that was full of love and life in the Holy Spirit. The same presence I felt in my bathroom. The same presence I felt at camp. I whispered, "God, you are amazing, and I thank you for your forgiveness, love and grace." Then I made a promise to God, which flowed out of me so naturally. "I will love you forever, and I will serve you with my life – *for all my days!*" I always felt guilty for ending the life of my baby, but today I was forgiven, and my guilt was gone. I sat grateful and humbled by the whole experience.

Rose brought me a glass of water, and I settled my mind back into the now. I went to collect Nathan. He didn't want to leave. It's always a good sign when kids love being where they are. I promised him we would come next Sunday.

As I drove home from church that afternoon, I had a strong feeling Alan was going to turn up at my house, and sure enough, he did. I don't know why I was so surprised. I had been praying all week for Alan to come and see me so that I could tell him all about my bathroom encounter with God, and my new-found peace. I was still getting used to sharing all my stuff with God, and then *things* happening.

Alan made his grand entrance. Tyres screeched, and burnt rubber filled the air as his V8 suddenly came to a halt in my driveway. His giant fist banged heavily on the front door, which I opened with great hesitation. He looked terrible and smelt like an old pub carpet. He was unshaven and bloated, which I suspect was from drinking too much alcohol.

Aggressively, he stated he wanted to see Nathan, who was now almost two. I feared Alan, but I had no right to stop him from seeing his son.

I stood aside and invited him in. Nathan immediately grabbed my legs and stayed very close to me. He was wary of this big, loud, and frightening man who he hadn't seen for nearly 12 months.

Anxiety rose within me, and I whispered a quick prayer. The Holy Spirit faithfully came with His incredible peace. Alan's powerful energy was always intimidating. He made me nervous at the best of times, but now his stance was hostile and defensive. The last time I saw him, he had walked out on me without a word. How do you pick up a polite conversation from there? I knew God was with me, and I wasn't afraid. I felt very calm as I made a pot of tea.

Alan noticed the church newsletter on the kitchen bench and said, "What's this, Emma, are you going to church now?" I knew he was smirking on the inside, insinuating I was weak and turning to religion for support.

But the Holy Spirit filled me, and my answer just flowed confidently out of my mouth, "Yes, I have only just started going. It's great, and Nathan loves it too!" As I spoke, the Spirit descended with more tangible presence and power. Alan became increasingly uncomfortable and fidgety. I knew he could feel the Holy Spirit, as well.

I asked him, "What's wrong? Why are you so uncomfortable?"

Alan replied defensively, "I don't know; it just feels like there are… ghosts in the air!"

Without thinking about what I was going to say, I launched into, "Well, that's because there is! It's the Holy Ghost! Do you know Alan, I have found Jesus, and He is so real? Jesus gives you the most amazing feeling." Then I made a bold statement. I straightened up with more confidence and said, "The *high* Jesus gives you, is a better *high* than any of the alcohol or drugs we ever took together." Alan just stared at me, not knowing how to respond. My heart softened towards him, and I continued with an invitation. "I am happy to tell you more if you want to know."

Alan seemed genuinely interested and said, "Yeah, sure, go ahead."

Thinking things through I replied, "Okay, would you like to stay for dinner? I have to feed Nathan soon and put him to bed, then perhaps we can talk." Alan agreed and even helped me in the kitchen. It felt strange. Part of me felt like he was an intruder and the other half as though we were still married.

I put Nathan to bed and said his prayers while Alan watched on. Our night-time routine was very different now, and Alan didn't say very much. I couldn't gauge what his impressions were, but as promised, we sat down on the lounge together, and I shared what had happened to me in my bathroom. Alan perked up and became surprisingly keen and proceeded to tell me he had a similar thing happen to him at a church once when he was 12.

As we shared, we pieced together that both our teenage spiritual experiences had happened at the same youth group, as he knew of Pastor Frank and Leanne. I didn't know if this was just another one of his lies, but everyone deserves a second chance – don't they?

I found myself offering Alan an olive branch. I spoke with tenderness and sincerity. "Maybe we could be a family again, but I can only see that happening *if* you become a Christian too." Living a Christian life was the only wholesome direction I wanted to take now for myself and Nathan. Alan seemed to be taking it all in.

He answered slowly, in a thoughtful tone while nodding his head, "I… think…I…do…want to become a Christian, Emma."

Shocked by Alan's answer, I started to panic as the reality of what I had just offered him dawned on me. *What was I saying? Am I stupid?* I didn't want to take him back! Alan was a thief, a liar, a cheat, a selfish manipulator, a con man, and a dominating, controlling narcissist! He possessed a natural ability to destroy everything and everyone around him, including me!

Anyway, I was quite safe. The reality of Alan becoming a Christian was highly unlikely. I figured – when he left tonight – I would probably *never* see him again. I was getting myself all worked up for nothing. I said goodbye to Alan, wished him well, and closed the door. *Nothing* prepared me for what was about to happen next.

CHAPTER 14

The Devil Himself

As soon as I shut the door, the hairs on my body stood tall, and I tingled. I walked into the living room, and an eerie presence followed me. It was so close I could feel its insidious hot breath burning the back of my neck. I was terrified. I turned around quickly to see what it was. Immediately the presence vanished. There was nothing there visible to my eye, but I knew a dark entity was somewhere in the house. Now, I was petrified.

I ran to Nathan's bedroom. He was fast asleep. I scooped him up in my arms, ran down the hallway into my bedroom, and locked the door. I had no idea how I thought closing the door would have helped – the evil not limited by solid matter. Nathan woke up in a daze.

I quickly placed him down on my bed and whispered, "It's okay darling boy; you can sleep with mummy tonight!"

My heart was racing. I got into bed and pulled the covers completely over both of us. I still had my clothes on, but I didn't care. I was panic-stricken. Nathan drifted back off to sleep. I held him tightly, not knowing what to do. I couldn't breathe. I lay there frozen with fear, my mind in turmoil. I could sense the evil, supernatural, heinous creature slithering closer towards us, so I cried out in prayer, *"God, please cover us with your protection from whatever this is!"*

I didn't know how it was possible, but it felt like Alan had left something evil behind from himself, or ushered it in, one of the two. A spiritual darkness, a foul entity. The sinister, demonic essence was sniffing us out. It was now just outside my bedroom. Then it turned and ran down the hallway as far as Nathan's door and turned again.

I sensed it was getting ready to run towards my room. Now, from under the covers – like a sixth sense – I could see it clearly, and I knew – *it was the devil himself!*

Its horny head was grotesque! Torn flesh hung off its face in dangling strips. Its beady eyes were glowing infra-red beams, and it stared right through into my soul. I saw its mouth dripping with black saliva and gnashing its razor brown, shark-like teeth in a snivelling, circular fashion. Its grey, slimy, lanky body swayed back and forth, teasing me with its horror.

I couldn't stop shaking. I squeezed my body, trying not to wet myself through absolute fear. I shut my eyes, but the image was as clear as anything. Then in a flash, it ran down the hallway towards my bedroom, but I also sensed a protective barrier. Somehow, it couldn't penetrate through the door.

When it realised it was blocked, it sent hundreds of gnashing teeth. They were able to reach me and appeared above my head. These were demons. They had no face, just razor-sharp teeth, snarling loudly and attempting to bite me like a swarm of piranha. I knew what I was experiencing wasn't in our earthly domain. I don't know how, but I could see into the spiritual realm. I hadn't asked for this. I didn't try to see it. I just did, and I didn't know how to escape it.

I tried to stay calm, and I prayed. I saw myself and Nathan in God's hands, and I focused on only that image. The demons delighted in their snarly taunts and continued in full force, but it soon became clear to me that no matter how hard they persisted, they couldn't touch us either. The protective barrier had covered Nathan and me. I focused on falling asleep. I held Nathan's warm body tightly in my arms, and eventually, I drifted off through sheer exhaustion from this evil, supernatural ordeal.

In the morning, when I awoke, it was gone. I thanked God over and over for His protection. I had no idea why that had happened to me, and I hoped I would never have any more encounters like that ever again.

But that evening, as dusk started to settle, I could feel the devil's presence sneaking around in the back garden wanting to come in again. I was petrified. I grabbed Nathan, my handbag and the car keys, and quickly raced to the car and drove over to Ronnie's house. I needed her to pray against this evil tormenting me for a second night.

I drove faster than I should have from the adrenaline pumping through my body. I frantically knocked on the front door hoping Ronnie was home. I didn't know what I was going to do if she wasn't. Thankfully the door opened, and as I stood in her lounge room, gushing forth the previous night's demonic events, Ronnie grabbed my hands and started shouting in what seemed like a different language. It was tongues. These mixed up sounds must have been what Jacky was talking about when we were at camp. I didn't understand it, but I didn't care.

If it worked – then go ahead! Shout to the heavens and get rid of it!

Ronnie's commanding prayer language subsided, and helplessly she looked at me and said, "Em, I can't do anymore! You need to go! Just thank God all the way home that it's gone."

I drove back at a much slower speed than when I left. I was so hesitant to go home, but as I drove past the park opposite my house, I saw an incredible sight. Again, I could see into the spirit realm. I saw 20 angels shining around the perimeter of my roof. The angels were at least ten feet high, and their bright display looked similar to candles on a birthday cake, burning in the darkness. Rays of glory were spearing out from them. *Immediately, I knew I was free from the evil presence.*

When Nathan and I walked through the door, more angelic beings greeted us. I could feel a celebration of victory all around me. Joining in with them, I danced around with Nathan, singing a little spontaneous song.

"We are safe, and we are free. God has given us the VICTORY! Angels all around tonight, shining forth their light so bright. We are safe, and we are free, God my Daddy, He's with me!"

Then I sensed God Himself settle on top of the roof. God was huge! His shoulders were massive, His hands powerful. Audibly, I heard His voice *Boom*. "SATAN! GO AWAY! STAY AWAY FROM MY CHILD! AND DON'T COME BACK!" God's sound in the atmosphere was louder than one thousand claps of thunder. The grotesque devil had been given its marching orders – never to taunt me ever again.

As I read my Bible, I could see the spiritual things that were happening to me were also in the scriptures. Reading these passages reassured me I wasn't going mad or making these occurrences up in my head.

I read, in Ephesians 6 verse 12, "For we wrestle not against flesh and blood, but against principalities, against powers, against the rulers of the darkness of this age, against spiritual hosts of wickedness in the heavenly places."

And in 1 Peter 5 verse 8, "Be sober, be vigilant; because your adversary the devil walks about like a roaring lion, seeking whom he may devour."

I understood we didn't just live in a physical world, but also a spiritual world as well – not unlike the vision I had on the bright and shiny road. The more I experienced God and read my Bible, the more I realised we truly exist in a world ruled by the devil and his demon hoards.

It is only when God Himself awakens our spirit – through Jesus and the Holy Ghost that we can see this phenomenon.

I was learning that because now my spirit is *born-again*, I *can* tune into God and this spiritual dimension. I was also aware that all Christians see, hear, and feel God differently. It was up to me – to seek out my relationship and communicate with God in a way that was right for me.

Reading the Bible, praying, listening to His quiet, still voice, singing, dancing, joining a church, were ways I could deepen my relationship with Him. God had an exciting kingdom of light for me to explore!

I wanted *everything* in this spiritual dimension that God could give me, including the gift of speaking in tongues. I saw the power of this heavenly language firsthand through Ronnie, and after what I had just experienced, I knew I needed it.

A tiny voice in my ear whispered, "*Tongues are of the devil.*" Years ago, when I was a little girl, I heard this declaration spoken at church. Of course, as a child, I had innocently believed their statement.

Now I was confused! If tongues were of the devil, why would God give the gift of this spiritual language to His believers? And, if they are of the devil, why does this powerful prayer language destroy the devil's atmosphere and his demon power? That didn't make sense!

I searched the scriptures to see what God's word said, and I read in Acts 2 verse 4, "And they were filled with the Holy Spirit, and began to speak with other tongues as the Spirit gave them utterance."

I prayed, "God, if tongues are of the devil – I don't want them. But *if* it is a powerful spiritual language that destroys the plans and strategies of the devil and his dark forces – then I do wish to have them, Amen!"

I waited for God's answer.

CHAPTER 15

Filled with Fire

I woke up the next morning with a strong urge to go to a traditional church in Fremantle, a city about half an hour from where I lived. I had never been into the church before, but I knew of it, and it was open to the public.

I also felt a strong sense to wear my grey dress. I remembered Jesus had worn grey when he sat at the end of my bed at the youth camp. He was full of humility. Maybe that colour was symbolic for me to reflect the same humble essence? I didn't know why – I just followed what I felt led to do.

I was learning that these intense feelings were God leading my spirit. It was one of the ways He communicated with me. Kind of like a gut feeling entwined with a warm, inner knowing sensation. My neighbour agreed to look after Nathan, and I set off to the church.

A magnificent, architecturally-designed stone building greeted me with open arched doors. I reverently stepped through onto a beautiful red carpet, which laid a welcoming track right down to the altar. Stained glass windows full of life and meaning reflected piercing colours of hope and promise. A five-foot eagle, made of solid brass, sat majestically on a carved wooden pedestal. Either side of it were palms releasing a serenity into the sanctuary.

My whole body tingled with a delicate excitement, and I knew I was about to have another spiritual encounter. Only one other woman was sitting on a pew; her head bowed in prayer. I sat right up the front and asked, "*God, why am I here?*" I closed my eyes. I sensed the Spirit of Jesus again in front of me, the same essence that appeared in my bathroom. I could hardly breathe.

I glanced back at the lady to see if she could see what was happening. *Was she able to sense this spiritual encounter? Was she aware that the Spirit of Jesus was standing here in front of me?* Her head still bowed down, so I assumed not.

I turned and faced Jesus again. Spirit to spirit, we talked. He asked gently. "*Do you want this gift?*"

I responded, "*Do you mean the gift of tongues?*"

"*Yes,*" Jesus replied.

"*So, they are not from the devil?*" I asked. I had to be sure.

"*No, they are a gift through the Holy Spirit.*"

I didn't quite know at this stage *how* I was going to get them, but I trusted Jesus with all my heart, so I said, "*Yes, I want them.*"

His hand reached out towards my closed mouth. A sensation like warm water flowed into me as though I was drinking a holy river. The unseen flow penetrated down into my belly, swirling around and around. *I knew I had just received the gift of tongues.* Jesus left, and I sat there, not knowing what to do next. It was all very well receiving them – now how did I get them out? I opened my mouth and pushed, but nothing happened. I did it again – still nothing. I left the church, thanking God for my newly acquired, angelic language, with another prayer request. "*How do I get them out?*"

Over the next couple of days, I pushed a few times here and there, trying to release the warm sensation I could still feel swirling in my belly. Still nothing. I persisted in prayer. "*God, please help me release them!*" Suddenly with a gush – out they came! So hard and fast, I couldn't stop them if I tried. A mixture of sounds and higgledy-piggledy words. Straight from the throne room in heaven. Woohoo! I have the heavenly language of angels, and the devil and his demons can't understand my prayers. Who said being a Christian is boring?

Walking daily with Jesus is the most incredible journey I have ever experienced in my life.

CHAPTER 16

What? Alan's Return

Exactly one week later, Alan arrived back and – *yes*, he had become a Christian and – *yes*, he wanted to be a family again. I was shocked beyond belief.

After the demonic experience I had in the house, I was incredibly wary of him.

But, if Alan had found Jesus, the Holy Spirit would have washed his life clean and pure too – right? Besides, I had offered him a second chance, so I hoped with his return and our newfound love for God, we would have a blessed and beautiful new beginning.

Welcome to the stage – Alan Janse! Reciting Bible scriptures and prayers with great enthusiasm, Alan was an explosion of Christianity. He had an unstoppable force to pursue *his call* he believed God had entrusted to him. God told him that he was to enter into church ministry and become a Pastor.

There was no denying God had touched his life. Alan was a dynamic preacher, a gifted worship leader, and he moved naturally with intense power in the things of the Spirit, although at times his delivery was harsh. I guess his insatiable pursuit for the things of God was better than his selfishness and lies, but apart from all the *seemingly righteous behaviour*, there was something about Alan that wasn't quite right. I just couldn't put my finger on it.

He was a lone ranger. I wanted to spend time with Alan, but he said to fulfil his call, he must spend hours in prayer by himself, which also is admirable, but our life was not in balance or harmony. We never talked or shared our faith, and we never prayed together. Alan and I were under the same roof living separate lives, once again.

I wanted to resolve and work through our betrayals when we were both unfaithful in our drug-addicted past. Perhaps even renew our vows. God had forgiven us, and it would be a rich experience for our relationship to declare our forgiveness to each other as well. I sensed we both needed healing, and it would give our marriage a fresh new start.

But Alan would not hear of it! Instead, he quoted the scripture in Philippians 3 verses 13 and 14, "but one thing I do, forgetting those things which are behind and reaching forward to those things which are ahead, I press toward the goal for the prize of the upward call of God in Christ Jesus".

Alan didn't want to share any process of restoration for our past and made it clear I was in the wrong by stirring up spiritual trouble, and I wasn't to mention it ever again.

Alan was determined to make his ministry happen for himself in any way he could. After spending days in prayer, he announced God told him to do the following two things. We had to sell our house – for the sake of the Gospel, and he had to go to Bible College for two years – at the best and most expensive campus in Australia. That meant we had to move interstate.

God had told him.

Who was I to argue with God? So, it started. God told Alan, Alan told me, and we did whatever Alan wanted. Nothing had changed. Alan was still dominating and controlling me, but now all under the guise of religion. The beautiful peace around me I had when I first found Jesus, was gone.

Here I was, walking on eggshells and trapped again. Trapped with what the church calls a wolf in sheep's clothing, and there was nothing I could do about it. Wolves are cunning and vicious by nature and devour the sheep. Alan's chameleon character charmed many people he encountered at church. He skilfully left them with his wool pulled firmly over their eyes. Other people never saw behind our closed doors. Alan made sure they always saw a perfect Christian couple.

I knew in my heart God had wanted me to give Alan a second chance, and I trusted God had a plan in what He was asking me to do, so I pressed on with the hope things would get better.

Scripture upon scripture, Alan showed me how God wanted me to act and behave to be the stereotypical Christian wife. His favourite was; submit and obey the husband. We never reviewed how a man valued and treated his wife, which is – love her, die for her, as Christ died for His church.

We quickly fell back into our old pattern of Alan being the puppet master; controlling, dictating, and pulling my strings. Alan's force was too strong for me. He always had a Bible verse to back up his requests. His unfair oppression spewed over Nathan and me daily. I had to smile and keep up appearances, but I was dreadfully unhappy and stressed. It was at this point I started suffocating internally, and my soul began to die.

As Alan frantically pursued his ministry, we became very involved in the church. All show and bravado, Alan paraded openly his charismatic call for all to see. People bowed down to him as though he was a mini-God, and Alan lapped up the applause. Our life was one big performance. I was behind the curtain and busy backstage, organising the perfect props for Alan's next scenes. He shouted his lines, and on cue, I acted accordingly. It wasn't a romance script. I lived in a chilling, horrific pantomime that was destroying me and out of my control.

My beautiful personal relationship with Jesus sustained me. Still, unfortunately, my anxiety condition that I had battled with all my life was flaring up and affecting my health again.

It was strange. Alan liked focusing on my ailing disposition. Somehow it made him feel superior, attending to my weaknesses. One anxiety trigger, in particular, was becoming more noticeable.

CHAPTER 17

The Wardrobe Door

All my life, out of habit, before I got into bed every night, I shut the wardrobe door tightly. The thought of the door being open, even a crack, still made me panic. I had been doing this subconscious routine every night for approximately 23 years. My wardrobe phobia highlighted I needed inner healing. No matter what prayer I prayed, or scripture I declared, I couldn't find a release. Pastor Frank, Isabelle, and Marcia, who were strong prayers in our church, offered to pray for me and this debilitating curse.

They all agreed and came to our home. We started by singing a few Christian songs which always ushered in the Holy Spirit and beautifully changed the atmosphere to a sweet, gentle presence.

With open hearts, our expectations grew for an encounter with God Almighty. Suddenly, a word dropped into me. Calamity! What a strange concept, I thought. What does that mean? I had heard of the cow-girl Calamity Jane when I was a child, but that was all.

We kept praying softly, seeking the Holy Spirit's guidance, then Isabelle said, "I see the wardrobe Emma, and inside it, there is so much fear. It is black, but I keep hearing this word, calamity!"

"Oh, my goodness," I said, "I got that word too!"

With that pearl of wisdom sent down from heaven, everyone gathered around me. Pastor Frank prayed against the word calamity, and for all the fear to go from inside the wardrobe and whatever dread it held for me. I felt God's presence strongly, although I didn't feel any different. I thanked everyone and believed in faith; something had shifted in the spirit realm, healing my phobia.

I went to bed, as usual, shutting the wardrobe out of a habit I had performed all my life. I thought nothing more about the wardrobe door or how the word calamity originated. As far as I was concerned, I didn't need to know the mystery, and I was glad to put it all behind me.

During my quiet times with God, I saw visions as if I was watching a black and white television. One time I saw a man in the church plotting to murder Pastor Frank. I phoned him immediately, and he confirmed I was the third person to tell him that news and the intercessors at the church would pray against that evil strategy assigned from Satan.

God was showing me more and more; I was fighting against these evil powers in the spirit realm. But God also showed me He is more powerful, and He is a God of miracles.

CHAPTER 18

It wasn't His Time

When Nathan was one year old, I gave him a whole egg in a milk drink. Immediately he struggled to breathe, and I rushed him to our local medical centre, where a nurse grabbed him from my arms. She quickly strapped an oxygen mask onto his face and gave him an adrenaline injection. The doctor said Nathan was highly allergic to eggs, and I must wait until he is seven years old before trying to give him one again and keep dairy food to a minimum.

Fast forward – Nathan was two; I had become a Christian and taken Alan back. We made sure our little boy followed his strict dietary requirements, and he hadn't had one flare-up.

We attended our church's Easter Camp, and without us knowing, Nathan had been eating vast amounts of ice-cream and Easter eggs with the other children. We didn't know because he didn't react. This amount of dairy should have set him off in an instant, but he was fine. I was amazed and thanked God because I had been praying for his healing. Nathan had so much fun with all the other children, but it tired him out, and when we arrived home, he went straight to bed.

The next morning Nathan was up bright and early, gobbled down his usual rice bubbles and milk, and went to play outside. In no time at all, he was gasping for breath so badly we knew we had to rush him immediately to the medical centre, but by the time I had grabbed my handbag and the car keys, Alan was shouting, "Emma, he's stopped breathing!"

I cried out immediately, "Oh God, help us, please!" I was hysterical. In the background, I heard Alan praying powerfully in tongues. I didn't know what to do. I phoned Pastor Frank to ask him to pray. No reply.

I telephoned Ronnie to ask her as well. No reply. I called Isabelle and the intercessors at the church. No reply. My attempts for help were futile. I was wasting precious time. I pleaded with God, "There is no one there to help us to pray!"

I felt God's warm still voice impress deeply on my heart, "Ask Me."

Of course! I fell to my knees, and through deep sobbing, I cried out with my direct request, "Please, God, please, don't let my baby die."

Now, Alan was shouting fiercely in tongues and holding Nathan's body high above his head in a desperate plea for God to grant us a miracle!

I was in a numb, dazed state of helplessness. More than 40 minutes had passed since Nathan had stopped breathing. I knew by now; my son would be dead, but Alan and I didn't stop our heart cry for healing. What else could we do? Where else could we go? God was our only hope for Nathan's life.

All of a sudden, an incredibly solid and weighty presence of the Holy Spirit came and filled the atmosphere of our little house. It was the glory cloud of God. It was so thick I had to push my body through it, as though I was walking against the wind. I forced my way to the lounge, sat down, and waited. There was nothing else I could do but to hold on to the mercy of God.

Alan stopped praying and came and sat down beside me. Holding Nathan's lifeless body in his arms, I looked at Nathan's little face. It was grey. The tangible presence of the Holy Spirit encapsulated us all. Alan turned to me and said, "God, just told me to blow on Nathan's face."

I looked at Alan and replied, "Okay… well… blow on his face!"

Alan blew with one steady, gentle and long breath all over Nathan's face. Nothing happened.

We waited. The cloud around us became even thicker.

We both sat quietly, not knowing what was going to happen next when the corners of Nathan's mouth quivered as though he was trying to smile. His face was still grey, but we knew God was in control and performing a miracle right before our eyes. Then, Nathan took a massive gulp of air, and his face changed to a shade of pink like a chameleon does to suit its surroundings. Nathan's surroundings were life and healing. Nathan had just received a miracle from God.

He was listless and frail for the rest of the afternoon. We sat with him on the lounge, patting his forehead with cold towels and giving him fresh orange juice to sip. We asked Nathan if he remembered anything. Even though he was only two years old, he could talk very well for his age.

He said Jesus came to him, took him by the hand, and they went to the park together. Jesus pushed him on the swing for quite a long time. Then Jesus told him he must go home to his daddy and mummy, and Jesus waved goodbye.

Alan and I were stunned as we listened, but we believed Nathan. He had no gain for himself to make anything like that up, and I am forever thankful to God – it wasn't his time.

Alan, of course, took this miracle to be a feather in his cap and declared now God had given him *a power ministry* and he could raise the dead. Alan became more prideful and arrogant if that was at all possible.

God was showing us what it was like to live our lives in the Spirit with Him. Little did I know it was my turn next.

Alan, myself and Nathan had just been to the Friday night outreach program held in the city. Our church provided raisin toast and a hot drink for people who came in off the street, and we shared with them the love and hope of Jesus. It had been a thriving, busy night.

It happened so quickly; no one saw it coming.

CHAPTER 19

The Accident

As Alan, Nathan and I left the church, Isabelle shouted across the car park. "Hey, you guys, come for coffee at my house before you drive home. Pastor Frank, Jason, and Claire are coming!"

Not that we needed any more to eat or drink. Our stomachs were full from all the cinnamon toast and hot chocolate, but it would be nice to chat and talk about the successful night.

Alan shouted back, "Okay, sounds good, Izzy. What's your address?"

"Just follow Jason," Isabelle shouted as she got in her car. Jason was already pulling out, so we followed promptly to form a five-car convoy.

Nathan was his usual chatty self and entertained us from his safety-chair in the back. Such a darling little boy always asking questions, and now he had discovered – why?

I couldn't wait to spend some time with Isabelle. She was so bubbly and happy – never short of a funny story, and we always had a girly giggle together. She radiated a loving warmth, and I always felt encouraged after being with her. I'm not sure if she knew how suppressed I was by Alan, but she stuck up for me if I had an opinion about anything.

The streets were not busy for a Friday night. I looked out my window, glancing at the shop fronts and their flashing neon signs as we drove along. I saw a couple of teenage boys hitchhiking on the side of the road. I thought they must be freezing as we were starting to get some cold nights. I remembered we needed to purchase wood for our fire. I turned to Alan and asked, "Did you…"

BANG!

Has someone just shot me in the head? That was my immediate thought, as I sat in the aftermath of the sudden impact. Still conscious but very stunned, I turned my head slowly towards Alan, who was still sitting in the driver's seat.

I could hear his faint voice, "Emma, can you hear me, can you hear me?"

I couldn't speak. *What just happened?* Alan got out of the car. I vaguely heard his muffled shouts to the others.

Everything was in slow motion, as sounds hummed around me. I wanted to scream, but nature's anaesthetic had numbed my body. I was in a state of shock. Warm blood, my blood, ran down the left side of my jacket, over my hand, and onto my jeans. I thought to myself; this is it – *this is my time to go!*

Instantly, a vision of Jesus appeared in front of me, and I heard His gentle, comforting words.

"I am with you!" Of course, you are Jesus, I thought to myself. You never leave me. It's Your promise. Jesus stood with His arms open wide, but I couldn't see His face. A shining glory covered it! I could only see His body from the neck down. His robe was ablaze with a blinding, white fire; I could barely look at Him. Jesus radiated an indescribable peace. He stood in front of me, gently saying over and over, "It's all right; I am with you." Behind Jesus were some enormous gates reflecting a shiny lustre promoting a royal sovereignty.

I looked beyond the gates, and I saw a bright green meadow, with trees that were so alive the leaves shimmered and moved with a glowing vibrancy. These were different from any trees I had ever seen. I saw flowers that had colours I had never seen before, or perhaps it was because the colours seemed to vibrate as well.

The air was fresh. It was clean and light, and there were streams of crystal-clear water that danced at the foot of very tall mountains that reverberated with a crescendo of joyful sound to the Creator. Actually, all of creation was singing praises to God Almighty. It was truly breathtaking.

The atmosphere was pure life itself. There was no sun or moon. No day or night. Just a beautiful ambience and serenity that, I assumed, people called heaven or the place you wait before heaven. I wasn't sure, but all I knew was this paradise was somewhere eternal my spirit would go to when it left my body.

I thought to myself; I am going here now. I was peaceful and calm. I had no fear at all – no regret for any part of my life. No sadness, knowing I would be leaving this earth. No pain, knowing I would leave my loved ones, nor any disappointment to not be able to wake up tomorrow to fulfil another day. I had a peace and excitement I would be leaving and going to this beautiful eternity with God my Father, and Jesus. I had no desire to stay on this earth; all I wanted was to live in this heavenly kingdom, forever.

I didn't know how to enter, so in my numbed state, I tried to push myself out of my body. I didn't leave, so I tried again, and again; nothing happened except for increasing the pain in my head. I tried one more time, but not as hard – and still, nothing. Jesus just stood surrounded by glory, giving me peace from His supreme glow. It was apparent to me now, I was not leaving my body, and I thought perhaps – maybe it's not my time.

By now, everyone in our convoy had stopped and were standing around our car. Isabelle opened my door and spoke to me. I heard the panic in her voice, "Emma, can you hear me, are you all right?"

I turned my head very slowly and replied in a slurred manner, "Yes, I'm fine; Jesus is here with me. I'm going to be okay."

Isabelle said, "That's wonderful, Emma, that Jesus is with you, but we are taking you to the hospital straight away!" I kept insisting I would be fine, almost arguing that I just needed to lie down. In Isabelle's humorous way of coping with the situation, she declared loudly, "Jesus, I need you too!"

As Isabelle undid my seatbelt, instantly, the vision of Jesus and heaven disappeared, and I crossed back into earth's reality. My head exploded with pain. Isabelle took the medical reins and organised for

Nathan to stay with a friend, while she and Alan delivered me safely into the hands of a plastic surgeon at the hospital.

And I needed help. The teenage boys had thrown a full can of drink at my window. It smashed through the glass at bullet speed, hitting my head, just below my left temple. It severed the top of my left ear – nearly entirely off – but not quite. The top part of my ear was hanging down by a thread. My left eye haemorrhaged and was swollen and bloodshot. The can then bounced off my head and smashed into the back window of our car at full force shattering the whole area. Small fragments of glass covered Nathan's head and body, filling up his car seat, but miraculously there was not a scratch on him. He never even cried. Had Jesus given him peace as well?

After a three-hour operation and 36 stitches later, my ear was sewn back onto my head.

The doctor did a fantastic job, and thankfully my hearing had not been affected.

There was a coincidence in this whole scenario. The doctor was a Christian, but she had seen too many horrific deaths over the years, challenging her faith in a loving God. She stopped going to church and hadn't prayed for a long time.

Under local anaesthetic, I shared my bathroom encounter and the genuine, powerful love of God with her. My experience touched her heart; she rededicated her life back to Jesus – right there at the operating table.

Why did that accident happen to me? So, I could share with her the love of God? Was it because I had prayed against the dark plans of evil? I got hit right under my temple, the place where I saw my visions. Whatever the reason, one thing I do know, God's ways are higher than our ways, and God's thoughts are higher than our thoughts. We can never work Him out, but we can trust He is sovereign, and He will bring good out of bad situations if we put our hope in Him.

Alan was annoyed my ear accident had happened. It slowed down his plans for his ministry. My parents were worried because of Alan's manic, obsessive, and selfish behaviour. He had now sold our house and was ready to take off to more abundant and greener pastures. Pastor Frank tried to encourage Alan to stay in the church so he could mentor him, but Alan did whatever Alan wanted. He had grand plans for himself, and no one was going to stop him.

CHAPTER 20

Following the Leader

Alan drove nearly non-stop from Perth to Sydney. Our whole lifestyle was manic and fixed at one speed – fast! One hundred miles an hour fast with Alan gripping the wheel. My legs spun like eggbeaters running to keep up with him. Pausing for a rest was not allowed. Life with Alan was exhausting and not enjoyable.

I fell pregnant again, and eventually, we welcomed to the world our beautiful baby girl, Hannah. I thanked God for another child to cherish. Nathan and Hannah were my life, my joy, and my blessings.

Life with Alan was hard when we lived in the West, but now, I was isolated. I had no friends and no family around me. Alan spent long hours at Bible College, and I spent my days typing up his assignments, looking after the children, and doing housework. While I was content being the homemaker, it was an incredibly lonely time. Our life only centred around Alan's plans.

Six months into Alan's two-year studies, he became a star student. Alan's natural abilities for ministry were outstanding, and he attracted attention wherever he went.

Teachers, elders and other ministers put Alan on a pedestal. They favoured him with many opportunities, even before other students who had been studying for a longer time. I couldn't understand how anyone else didn't see Alan's selfish agendas and ulterior motives. His charisma had blinded them. After only six months of Bible College, Alan was offered the senior position to pastor a church in Queensland.

Being young Christians of only two and a half years, we were very inexperienced in the ways of God, and any form of ministry. Alan had just turned 26, and his character certainly hadn't been tried and tested for a leadership position. I felt it was far too much, and way too soon for both of us, but nothing was going to stop him, and anything negative I projected, Alan told me Satan had possessed my thoughts.

Cracks were appearing in my health, and I was on the verge of burn-out, but Alan scolded me for *my* selfishness and my lack of concern for saving lost souls. We waited on the confirmation for Alan's acceptance to pastor the church. It took a few weeks to process Alan's new ordained role. In that time, my health had suffered more setbacks. I developed migraines and insomnia, but Alan denied me any care or consideration. His one focus was the ministry.

The magnitude of what was ahead caused me to have a break-down, and my mother immediately flew over. She nursed me for two months and looked after the children, and although I was far from recovery, Alan was not going to dismiss the position for pastoring the church.

As soon as Alan could arrange things, he forfeited Bible College, and after packing up our house, we frantically set off into the unknown territory of ministry. Serving as a Pastor's wife was the last thing I felt capable of being, and I always felt like I was one small step away from having another breakdown.

When Alan took over the church in Queensland, it was a congregation of approximately 80 people. The church didn't take long to grow. Word spread around town; there was a new dynamic Pastor on the block. Alan's charisma enabled him to preach the Bible in a way that was exciting for the listener. People were drawn in by his charm, and very quickly, the flock had tripled in size in a few months. New faces were showing up every week, and many were giving their lives to Jesus, getting healed from illnesses and delivered from spiritual strongholds. Every Sunday, the services exploded with the Holy Spirit's fire.

Other ministers were asking Alan for his strategies and blueprint techniques for church growth. Some flew from other countries to sit at his feet and glean for tips for growing their churches too. This global attention swelled his pride, and in his mind, made him even more superior and spiritually powerful than anyone else.

Everything Alan did, he did for himself, not for God. He was the driver of *his* glory train. Alan spent thousands of dollars on theology books, tailor-made anti-crush suits, and spared himself nothing. He needed the latest gadgets on the market, and of course the most expensive. His extravagant spending was always justified. The money from the sale of the house was quickly dwindling.

Alan took the children and me to the op-shop for our needs. Don't get me wrong. I love a good op-shop. It was just the way Alan treated us that upset me. With insignificance and disregard. Somehow this existence was all too familiar. I lived with a king who dined on a lavish banquet while Nathan, Hannah, and I scraped up sparse cooked rice while sitting on prickly hessian bags.

Our neglect was not visible. It was little by little and bit by bit; subtle, almost unseen to the onlooker.

The children and I were all suppressed by Alan regarding – what we thought, what we ate, what we wore, and what we watched on television. Alan scrutinised everything through his selfish filter, so no surprises, we were last on the list.

Now the puppet master had three puppets to manipulate. Nathan and Hannah had only one chance to obey Alan and do it right. If not, he would discipline them very harshly to the point of abuse backed up with a scripture from the Bible.

Alan continued to weave his thick, black threads into our lives. His words were needle-point sharp and extremely painful as he pricked us deeply. The pattern that was emerging day after day was frightening and ugly.

Nathan was five, and Hannah was two. Alan couldn't interact with Hannah because of her age. He had no interest in any form of child's play. He purposely ignored her and went weeks without any interaction. Some may see that as sad. It was for her blessing. Thankfully,

Hannah missed out on Alan's harsh discipline. Nathan, unfortunately, copped it all.

There are far too many past sad memories to tell, but I will share a few of our unfair life dynamics.

Nathan idolised Alan and begged his daddy many times to throw the ball and simply be a father. Alan gave the usual excuses of having to do ministry work or being too tired.

If at any time Alan was forced to play catch with Nathan, in front of family or friends, to keep up appearances, Alan put on his; *I'm the world's greatest dad act.* When nobody was looking, his throws changed to hard and fast. He made it impossible for Nathan to catch the ball.

Alan would pull Nathan aside and say, "When you are a bit older, we will play son, you are just too young to catch the ball yet!"

Nathan, in his childlike nature, would reply, "Okay, I can't wait till I am older! I love you, daddy, and when I grow up, I want to be just like you!"

Alan coached his son by saying, "Well, go and be a good boy then and get daddy another drink!"

It didn't matter what Alan did, in Nathan's eyes, his daddy was the best! Alan was his idol, and he tried his hardest to please his daddy at every request.

Alan took the drink and said, "Don't go too far, son. Daddy will want another one soon."

I saw Alan's interaction with his son, and I was reminded of the song by Harry Chapin: Cat's in the Cradle. I wondered when Nathan grew up and realised for himself who Alan really was if he would ever want to be like his dad.

What I am about to write next is quite disgusting. I thought long and hard if I needed to share it, and part of me didn't want to. But how can I portray Alan's warped behaviour and character if I don't talk about the things we had to live with? I will try not to go into explicit detail.

We had two little Dachshund dogs. A boy called Clive, and a girl named Maggie. They were adorable. Very naughty, as these sausage-dogs are; they chewed holes in the furniture and our shoes. All the usual things that dogs do. And occasionally, at times, they would hump your leg or anyone else's leg who came to visit. With acute embarrassment, I would promptly growl at their feral behaviour.

But it wasn't their fault. Alan encouraged them to have an unsavoury sexual appetite, offering them his arm or leg and brought them to full arousal. Then he laughed and stated animals needed relieving just like human beings do, and he was doing them a favour.

It made me feel sick. Alan was a Minister of Religion, and this was bordering on bestiality.

I asked him many times, "Alan, don't you think this is wrong?"

He replied, "Stop judging me, Miss High and Mighty! You over-dramatise everything. Stop being a super-spirro!" Super-spirro was a term used in the church to make fun of a spiritual person who is over-the-top with religious enthusiasm.

Calling me a super-spirro diverted any accountability. Alan's criticism chipped away at me steadily. Alan was right. I was wrong. My heart to please God and be a good Christian wife was my aim, so I dutifully obeyed.

The day Nathan turned three, Alan crowned him chief dog-poop-picker-upper, as though this was some elite status. Normally, I would do it, but I was pregnant and wasn't allowed near animal faeces – and Alan just didn't want to do it.

Don't get me wrong; I think it's imperative to give your children chores. Nathan, as usual, would do it with great effort, wanting to do an excellent job for his daddy. But Alan's narcissistic attitude gave him great pleasure in teasing his little boy.

If mocking jeers such as, "It's a bird, it's a plane, no it's poo-man," were not enough to ridicule Nathan, Alan would take centre position on a chair on the lawn with his guitar and make up a song.

While Nathan was scooping, Alan would chime, "He's picking up poo, he's good at it too, Nathan the poo-man. Smelly brown poo, he smells like it too, Nathan the poo-man."

Verse after verse Alan's subtle bullying mixed with a glib, sarcastic sound, not only made him feel superior but would also seep into Nathan with a degrading penetration.

Nathan craved Alan's approval, but nothing Nathan did was ever good enough.

Once, Nathan exclaimed with excitement, "Daddy, come and look, I've tidied my room and put the books back on the shelf neatly like you asked."

Whenever Alan interacted with the children, I always held my breath.

Nathan stood proudly, waiting to impress his father. Alan walked straight over to the bookshelf.

"What's this?"

Alan's manner was like a strict army officer.

"What did I say, Nathan, about these books?"

Timidly Nathan spoke. "You said, Daddy, to put them in order from big books to small books. Look, I did it!"

Nathan's face glowed with innocent pride as Alan ran his fingers over the tops of the stacked books. They were done very well for a four-year-old.

"Look at this."

Alan glared.

"And this!"

A couple of them were not in height order by about half a centimetre. With one swift action, shelf after shelf, Alan swooped them all onto the floor. They bounced in all directions and were more mixed up than ever.

"Do them again! Are you stupid? I said perfect order, perfect height, perfect, perfect, perfect!"

Alan shouted forth his demands.

"I want them done in five minutes, and if they are not perfect, you will get the stick!"

Nathan of course panicked and started putting the books back as fast as he could. He knew it would take longer, and he didn't want to get the stick.

Alan didn't always use the stick. He whipped out the belt and buckle, or at times, a cricket bat to hit Nathan into line.

Alan would say, spare the rod, spoil the child, and God had personally told him that the larger the rod, the less spoiled the child would be.

God had said.

Although this scripture is in the Bible, I saw the meaning differently. The shepherd's rod is a tool used for instruction and protection. A loving shepherd uses it softly and carefully with a tender heart to gently guide each little lamb and correct its steps from going astray.

Alan delighted in the correction of the physical kind, so he twisted the scripture to the context he wanted. I tried everything to stop Nathan from being beaten again and again and for minor occurrences. Alan would pull him and push me, drag Nathan behind closed doors, and keep me locked out. The sounds of Nathan screaming for his daddy to stop will be etched into my memory forever! I felt helpless, crying out to God to make Alan – just stop.

But Alan never did.

The suppressed abuse in Nathan came out during his sleep in the form of night terrors. He would stumble around the house, sleepwalking with his glazed eyes wide open, screaming, crying, and shaking uncontrollably. Alan would shout at Nathan, demanding him to be quiet! It was an impossible request as the nightmare had Nathan trapped. Alan would grab Nathan and slap him across the face trying to snap him out of it; only this heightened the hallucinations and distress.

Alan would get frustrated very quickly, and go back to bed, leaving Nathan still locked in his terror.

"See if you can sort him out, Emma," Alan would say, "I've had enough! I'm sick of Nathan waking me up every night. This behaviour has to end!"

I would take my beautiful little innocent boy and wrap my arms around him. I whispered in his ear soft promises of love and blessing using tender words of comfort as they came to me. I sang my prayers to soothe his soul, my fingertips stroking lightly over his forehead to release the tension. His little arms were clinging to me in sheer desperation as I rocked him gently. Singing calmed him back to sleep and worked every time. Unfortunately for Nathan, they were now becoming a nightly event.

Then my turn came. Lists of scriptures Alan gave me to read over and over about submission, sacrifice, and obedience to the husband. This one was his favourite: "Ephesians 5 verse 22 – Wives, submit to your own husbands, as to the Lord. For the husband is the head of the wife, as also Christ is head of the church".

After a while, I was a timid, sub-subservient Pastor's wife. I was too scared to say or do anything that would displease my husband or even worse; discredit his ministry, as Alan said God would be displeased with me. I didn't dare upset Alan. But no one else ever witnessed how he treated his children or his wife.

Alan's evil force affected my health more and more. I now lived in a state of continual anxiety, depression, and fatigue. The demands on me as a mother and Pastor's wife had drained me, and after a year of ministry, I couldn't do it anymore. I was utterly burnt-out and had nothing to give anyone. I desperately wanted to leave Queensland and return home, but I had to stay. Alan became furious if I mentioned anything of the sort.

Day after day, I had to keep giving from a flame that was no longer alight, and as I focused on my duties as a pastor's wife, my health kept deteriorating. The pressure to keep wearing my mask of happiness was destroying me. I cried out to God to help our marriage, and every time, I remembered my wedding vows. For better, for worse, in sickness and in health, until death do us part. I prayed God would give me the strength so I could be faithful to my commitment. But no matter how determined I was, things never changed.

It was at this point I had my second breakdown. Mother flew over again to look after me but could only stay a few weeks. After she left, I was in deep despair. All I could do was pray the footprints poem and ask God to carry me. There seemed to be no light at the end of this very long, dark, confusing tunnel.

Our parishioners were very worried about me. Alan told them the devil was making me sick to pull down his powerful and anointed ministry God had given him. Then Alan scolded me for allowing the devil to come into my life and make me sick. He insisted it was because I wasn't using my scriptures enough, and my faith was weak. Then other Pastors, their wives, and people in the congregation started telling me I was allowing the devil to make me sick because I wasn't using my scriptures enough, and my faith was weak. They were becoming Alan's puppets too. His charisma was very impregnable.

I felt like I was going crazy! Maybe I was, perhaps they were right? Maybe my faith was weak? I was so confused. I had no one to confide in and share my tortured life. There was no one I could go to for help. I was trapped. All I could do was pray.

The wolf was slowly, but surely, devouring this little sheep. Alan's compulsive lying was back in full force, and over time his lies infiltrated into the church. I guess it's hard to cover every deceitful track when you have paved so many as Alan had.

There were thousands of dollars of church funds missing, and rumours of pastoral visits with single ladies that lasted much longer than they should have. There were now large cracks in his character when he preached and the way he behaved. The elders were bound by duty to hold him accountable.

The church board approached Alan for investigation, but he twisted and turned situations around to suit himself. But they had enough witnesses and whistle-blowers to expose him and were going to proceed with the official application for personal review and audit. Of course, he kept this all from me. I had no idea any of this was going on.

Suddenly, out of the blue, Alan was concerned for my health and wellbeing and told me he had resigned. I was shocked. Alan putting me first? That had never happened. He told me his resignation was a declaration of his love for me. God told him we had to leave and go home, so I could rest and get well. Maybe my prayers for Alan to love and care for us were finally being answered after all?

We had no finances, according to Alan, so my parents yet again injected more funds to help with our return. I had never seen him in such a mad panic organising our departure. I was overwhelmed; he cared for me this much.

We had our last church service. Alan announced his public resignation to a shocked congregation. He shared it was because of my health issues that we were leaving. Everything felt wrong, and while our parish was genuinely understanding, I left church that day feeling like the biggest failure, to God, the church, and as a wife and mother.

In the morning, Alan filled the car with our belongings, keen to set off. One of the elders came to our house just as we were leaving, and he was angry. Alan shouted at the children and me to get in the car, and we obeyed promptly. Goodness knows what was going on, but it wasn't the first time I had witnessed an elder not seeing eye to eye with Alan. Their arguing escalated and nearly turned into a punch up.

With full strides, Alan got in the car, slammed the door and started the engine. The elder followed in hot pursuit. He hadn't finished with their altercation. Alan put the car in reverse and spun the wheels, creating a thick black dust which floated down all over the angry elder, and covered our vehicle. With a fierce glare, the elder shouted at my closed window.

"I DON'T THINK YOU KNOW EMMA, EXACTLY THE TYPE OF MAN YOUR HUSBAND IS!"

I was bewildered.

"Oh, my goodness Alan, what's happened? What does he mean?"

Alan snapped back with his ever-ready fast reply.

"He's just jealous of me Em because I'm such a powerful man of God and have a dynamic ministry ahead of me. He has been spreading lies about me, so if you ever hear anything on the grapevine – it's not true."

Knowing Alan was capable of lies, I didn't know what to believe. Living in a state of confusion was normal for me. As Alan sped away, I turned and looked back to see the black dust cloud following us. I had an instant evil-foreboding this was a prophetic omen of things to come. But right now, I couldn't care. I was depressed and exhausted on every level. The children and I were going home, and for me, that was a small light flickering ahead in the darkness.

It was beautiful to get back to the West Coast. I had missed Mother and Dad so much. I knew I could count on their love and support for myself and the children. I never told them anything negative about Alan as I was mindful of being a dutiful Christian wife. I didn't have to, though. They saw through his masquerade long ago.

My parents let us stay with them until we rented a house. We had nothing. Alan had spent every cent from the sale of our home, and I had no idea what on. Alan justified everything as usual.

And, Alan's concern for my anxiety and exhaustion was short-lived. I had been naïve to believe this was going to be his turning point to be a loving husband. We quickly got back into the groove of Alan living for Alan and doing anything to promote himself back onto his church pedestal.

As far as the children and I were concerned, Alan's tomorrows never came, and he always broke his promises. His words were never black or white, and we lived within a hazy grey, similar to the blurred existence in my childhood when I couldn't see. His lies and dysfunction made everything cloudy. Instead of building our family life on a strong foundation of love and honesty, the children and I sank daily in a quicksand of his narcissistic neglect.

Alan disregarded my burn-out, and we soon got back into the flow of busy church life. Desperate to return to ministry, one of Alan's acquaintances opened a door for a part-time position as Assistant Pastor in his Assembly. Working two days a week didn't provide enough money to survive, so Alan's brother, who worked at Crown Casino, also hustled a manager's position for Alan. Visible to everyone, this place of frivolous excitement and gambling was not cohesive with the purity of a Minister of Religion, but Alan convinced everyone we needed the money. And of course, God said it was fine.

I fell pregnant again, and soon I held in my arms another beautiful baby girl, Sarah. This pregnancy had been exhausting, but I was girded with an inner determination to press on. My children were my sole purpose for enduring another day. With the extra demands on me from Alan's part-time ministry and now his newly appointed casino position, I dragged myself along with a fake smile and pretended to do life. We still appeared to be the perfect Christian family that everyone looked up to, and to Alan, that was all that mattered.

Day after day, I cried out to God to hear my distress and heal my mind, my body and my marriage. Heaven was silent, apart from the overwhelming sense God loved me. He reassured me He knew all things and was working everything for good. I was simply to trust Him.

CHAPTER 21

Psalm 23

One Sunday after church, we arranged an afternoon tea for a visiting Prophet. He was a well-respected Minister on the world stage and spoke with authority and accuracy. I caught the Prophet staring in my direction, and then quite unexpectedly, he walked over to me.

"God has a word for you, my dear," he said.

His direct approach took me by surprise, though I felt incredibly privileged. I sensed the Holy Spirit's presence strongly emanating from him, and the hairs on my arms tingled. I knew God had sent him, and I looked at him with great curiosity and trepidation.

He proceeded to quote from memory Psalm 23.

"The Lord is my shepherd; I shall not want. He makes me to lie down in green pastures. He leads me beside still waters; He restores my soul. He guides me in paths of righteousness for His name's sake. Yea, though I walk through the valley of the shadow of death, I will fear no evil, for You are with me, Your rod and your staff, they comfort me. You prepare a table before me in the presence of my enemies, You anoint my head with oil, my cup runs over, surely goodness and mercy shall follow me all the days of my life, and I will dwell in the house of the Lord forever."

He held my hands and looked compassionately into my eyes.

"This Psalm is for you. I'm sorry to say that there *is* something terrible ahead of you, but God wants to tell you. FEAR NOT! He will bring you through it!" As he talked to me, he checked to see where Alan was. It was as though he instinctively knew he didn't want Alan to hear.

I nodded out of politeness and respect, but internally I was screaming! WHAT! I had never heard such a horrible word of prophecy! God wouldn't tell me THIS! God's predictions are encouraging; they give you hope, not anxiety! How could I be happy to receive this?

I smiled and thanked him, but I wrestled with his words for two weeks. The more I fought it, the more the Prophet's words intensified as truth within me.

Of course, I had no idea what something terrible meant, and it was only natural I didn't want it to be right, but the conviction in my spirit as to what he said was real and took me to a place where I finally had to surrender to it. I knew something dark and devastating was going to unfold ahead of me. And whatever it was, I knew God would be with me every step of the way.

Life had left me some signs, and I sensed the *terrible* had something to do with the black cloud I saw the day we left our church to come home. I sensed, whatever it was, it could be potentially life-destroying, but the Prophet gave me two words along with my Psalm 23 prophecy. Two words from God to – FEAR NOT!

It was frustrating because my gut instinct kept nudging me. Something was not right, but until whatever this was came into the light, I just couldn't see it. But I knew my world wouldn't stay in darkness forever. Eventually, a new day dawns, and the sun shines. Because of this fact, I had hope and faith.

I prepared myself for what was ahead, and I knew if I trusted in God, I would be okay.

Alan's dictatorship became more severe. Our controlled lifestyle increased to a strict regime to the minute. The children must be bathed, fed, and put to bed by 6.00 pm every night. I was only permitted to tuck them in and say their prayers for one minute each. Of course, God said this was to be the routine. Alan glared at me through the doorway to their rooms if I went over time, shouting a distant half-hearted goodnight to his children. Alan never spent any time with them reading or playing. Every day he was too busy living his separate agenda.

I discovered some of my gold jewellery had gone missing.

I asked Alan, "Have you seen my earrings, bracelets and necklaces that my parents gave me? I can't find them."

I was used to him firing scriptures at me instead of having a conversation, so his reply didn't surprise me.

"Emma, if you read in 1 Peter 3 verse 3 and 4 – God says, 'do not let your adornment be merely outward – arranging the hair, wearing gold, or putting on fine apparel. Rather let it be the hidden person of the heart, with the incorruptible beauty of a gentle and quiet spirit, which is very precious in the sight of God'".

I was confused and answered with a frown. "Yes, I know that scripture is in the Bible – but I can't find them. I have always kept them in this box, and they are not here."

Alan became increasingly annoyed with me.

"Use your brains, Emma, where do you think they are?"

I had no idea.

"I don't know," I replied, "but I will be upset if something has happened to them. Do you think someone has stolen my jewellery?"

"You are so dense! I've hocked them at the pawnbroker. I needed some money." His tone was emotionless as if it was his right to sell them.

Alan was always hocking our things, but I couldn't believe he had taken my jewellery. My reply was quiet and slow.

"I can't believe you have hocked my precious things!"

Alan was ready, scripturally loaded, to fire another one.

"Philippians 2 verse 14 – 'Do all things without complaining and disputing'. Emma, do you need reminding?" Alan followed with his signature dominant glare.

Whenever Alan said, "do you need reminding," it meant, that's enough now if you know what's good for you, let me do what I want to do. Get back in your box and let me shut your lid.

Alan never hit me. He didn't have to. I always did what he said. I would have an anxiety attack just at the thought of standing up to him. His daily emotional and psychological punches left me with internal bruises. I was trapped in this marriage and trapped within myself. After years of suppression, I was barely alive.

I can't emphasise enough, I did try to speak up for myself about his unreasonable mannerisms and keeping me in line with the scriptures, but it was no good. The Bible has millions of scriptures, and I was put back in my box with every single one of them. As magicians pull rabbits out of hats, Alan pulled verses out of the Bible to suit his situation.

Hocking my jewellery had hurt me more than anything, but I was grateful for one thing. My Grandma's wedding ring was miraculously somehow still in the corner of the box. I put it on my finger, where I knew it would be safe, fearing nothing in my life was safe anymore.

CHAPTER 22

A Dark Valley

Alan's behaviour became even more chaotic if that was possible. Always in a rush, he couldn't stand still for one second and lived as though he was standing on hot coals. I never knew where he was or where he went. There was no point even asking because it was always a quick-fire answer I knew was a lie.

Our family structure was manic with no foundational security. Any money that came in quickly fell through the holes in Alan's pockets. Alan updated our car every few months. We moved to a different house every six or twelve months when the lease was up. We lived as though we were on the run from someone chasing us.

Mobile phones had just entered the market. Alan purchased one and disconnected our landline. His reasons were it was cheaper just to have one phone. That's very true, but that meant I had none.

The postman stopped delivering letters to our house. I thought it was strange that we suddenly didn't get mail anymore. I found out eventually Alan had taken out a central box at the post office. His reasons were always – God said.

We had only one car, and I had no access to transport. I couldn't go anywhere, and no one could contact me to arrange a visit. Alan said he had purposefully done all this so I could have peace to get well from my anxiety and exhaustion. It was his way of caring for me.

I didn't know at the time that one of the things a narcissist will do is *gaslight* his victim. They keep them far away from family and friends. Because we had to move back to the West, this tactic of isolation was Alan's next best thing.

Keeping up appearances was paramount. The children and I obeyed our strict orders in how we were to behave, and we faithfully attended church every Sunday as a smiling, happy family. Behind my mask lived a functioning zombie, while Alan pranced around the stage, shouting and preaching his catchy sermons, soaking up the accolades and compliments afterwards. Alan lived for being noticed and made sure I was not!

The children and I had lived in this suppressive dysfunction for six years now. I didn't know how much more I could take. I was now a fragile shell of a woman. Every morning I woke up foggy and exhausted, but I pushed myself to walk the children to school every day. Most afternoons we went to the park opposite our house. We spent a lot of time at the pond feeding the ducks. This simple outing was the highlight of my life and a small escape to normality. I loved being with my children.

Despite living in Alan's hellhole, there were glimpses of heaven when God would shine down into my life. Amidst the unfairness and abuse in our lives, the children and I had our bond of love Alan could never destroy, no matter how hard he subtly tried.

At times Alan disappeared for days. He said he was working double shifts at the casino or helping people in need at the church. Alan controlled everything, and I had no car, no phone, no money, and little to no food, but he was careful not to let us starve.

When he announced he was going away for long periods, he made sure we always had a jumbo-sized box of Weetabix and boxes of milk. The children and I ate Weetabix for two or three days in a row for breakfast, lunch, and dinner. I could never say to Alan we had nothing to eat. The grey truth was, we did.

Many times, I asked him, "Can the children and I perhaps have something other than Weetabix?" But our menu never changed.

The standard answer for any of my requests was, "We don't have any money." End of story. Funny though, Alan found hundreds of dollars to spend on himself.

After a while, I just gave up and tried to make the most of what I did have. Fighting for my freedom was too exhausting.

Anyway, if I did request anything, now I could answer myself with the applicable scripture, I heard them all so often.

When Alan eventually came home, he was puffed up in his pride, boasting of the beautiful world-class evenings he was having while at work in the casino, the live shows and concerts he got to see, and the luxury five-star food he was eating, provided on his meal tickets. It was as though he delighted in taunting the children and me in any way he could.

It was very apparent we were living separate lives, but he was always home for Sunday to take the church service and preach his sermon. In front of his religious peers, he had to appear to have it all together. It was just not right.

His chameleon existence, with one foot in the casino and one foot in the church, continued strongly behind our closed doors. He covered his tracks and spun many fanciful stories to everyone to make sure it stayed that way.

I felt like I was in one of those double-life sick, twisted movies. Alan's favourite line in our thriller was, *I've got everything under control!* This phrase meant many things. Don't you dare get involved. Don't ask questions. Don't you have an opinion. Don't say any more on the matter. My acting cue was to nod, smile, and say nothing. If I didn't, Alan shouted in annoyance that God would be angry with me, and now – I would even go to hell!

Sociopaths have a calculated style of brainwashing. They use the very things you love to ignite their power.

It's funny how sometimes you don't know, but you just do. Alan walked into the house one day and went straight into the bathroom.

Without even thinking about it, I blurted out, "Alan, you are having an affair!"

They didn't even feel like my words, but they had come from my mouth, *and*, with such conviction. I had no proof, no logical reason to say such a thing, but I had said it. Alan swiftly came out of the bathroom, wiping his mouth with a towel. He glared at me. I could tell he was angry.

"What on earth are you talking about, Emma? I went and washed my face because I just ate a pie and sauce, and I wanted to be fresh so that I could kiss you. Are you suggesting I have been with another woman?"

I froze. Why did I say that? I knew better than to challenge him. I stared blankly and said nothing!

Instantly he fumed.

"How dare you, Emma, accuse me of such a thing. I am a man of God and married to you.

How dare you say something like that!" He started pacing around in circles, throwing his arms up in the air.

"You are crazy, Emma! The devil has you tied around his little finger."

He mimicked me in a sour girl's voice, "*Alan's having an affair, and I'm letting the devil make me crazy!* Grow up, Emma. You are insane. You have a mental disease! In here."

He tapped his head, "In your brain, you are mental!"

Maybe I was losing my mind? My brain *was* always foggy, and my life continually hazy. I had no idea why I said that. Whether I was right or wrong, I had undoubtedly pushed Alan's buttons. What was I thinking? I knew full well the repercussions of Alan's wrath, and the last thing I wanted to do was to stir him to anger.

Of course, I retreated. I was shaky, tearful, and drained.

I surrendered to him, "I don't know why I even said that Alan, I'm sorry! Every day, I don't feel well, and my mind plays tricks on me again and again. I'm sorry, please forgive me."

Alan was expressionless as he walked over to me. I felt the power raging within him, and I was frightened. He was so unpredictable I never knew what was coming at me next.

He took hold of my hands and slipped straight into prayer. It rolled off his tongue with a professional Pastors' eloquence.

"Our Loving Father in heaven, you see Emma in her sickness and troubled mind, and I ask you to show her how much I love her. Show her I would never be with another woman apart from her. We are married in your sight, and I love and respect her with every part of my being. Strengthen the cords that bind us together in marital harmony and bring peace to her mind and show her I would never cheat on her, never be unfaithful to her. She is the only woman for me – now and forever. Bless our marriage! In Jesus' precious name. Amen!"

His words lulled me into a numb existence of hopeless calm. "Now Emma," he said as he jumped up quickly, "I'm busy, and I've got church stuff to do!"

He turned around and walked out the door.

I tried to feel peaceful, but inner turmoil swirled inside my body and my mind. Oh! And he never kissed me.

Now, Alan was never home during the week, as he rented a hotel room at the casino. He told me, *just by looking at me*, it made him feel less of a man and husband. Alan said it was because his prayers couldn't make me well, and I made him feel angry and a failure, both at once. I was a distraction he didn't need, and God wouldn't want him to waste his energy on someone who didn't want to learn their scriptures and help themselves. He said I had brought my years of health issues upon myself.

The following week Alan had come home to sleep, which was unusual, and three nights in a row, I was woken up by strange sounds coming from the television. It was porn. Of course, I questioned his actions. He was doing a series of teachings in the church on holiness and purity. It wasn't right! Alan, furious, rebuked me for my judgement. He twisted his way around this, and once again, I found myself apologising. His insipid, dominating suppression was crippling me.

CHAPTER 23

The Shadow of Death

From here, I went downhill rapidly.

Trapped in deep depression and confined to bed, my memory was quickly fading to the extent of not remembering my name or my children. I couldn't talk without weeping profoundly. Each day, panic attacks constantly reoccurred, some lasting hours.

Painful headaches gripped my mind like a tightened vice. Anxiety raged, and I couldn't stop crying internally.

As the darkness of night approached, an evil foreboding enveloped my whole being, with the turmoil of yet another dark sleepless night.

Alan had to take the children to school. Interrupting his schedule made him furious. He made it clear I disrupted his pastoral freedom and casino playtimes.

The headaches upgraded to a migraine that exploded in my head. Alan stood over me, holding eight Panadol in his hand.

"Here, Emma, you need to take these," he said forcefully.

Something inside me screamed this was far too many.

I spoke in a weak quiet voice, "Alan, it's too many all at once."

"Rubbish," Alan replied. "Here, look on the box; you are allowed eight per day. You'll be fine."

Besides, God had told him it was okay for me to take eight at a time. I only ever saw Alan's outstretched arm holding the designated eight, white large pills. I had lost track of time, so I didn't know how often he was feeding them to me. With every pill I swallowed, I said a silent prayer for God to protect my kidneys and liver.

Breathing was now an effort. I lay in bed wondering, *if I just stopped taking air into my body, I could quietly die, and then I would escape this torment.* The only way I can describe the way I felt was – my mind was sleeping, in a coma, while my body was fully awake.

One day a couple in the church came to see if I was okay. I hadn't attended for months, and they were concerned. Alan convinced them I had allowed the devil to control me. I heard him saying, "We need to convince the elders to place Emma into a mental home."

Their reply was, "Absolutely Alan; we are so sorry to hear Emma has let this happen to herself. It must be so hard for you and the children. We will support you to make sure this goes ahead."

Shocked beyond belief at what I had just heard, I lay in bed, helpless and weak, listening to Alan hood-wink these people to help him plan my fate.

After they left, Alan came into the bedroom, pacing around the bed, quoting scriptures.

Angrily he shouted without pausing, "Are you listening to me? You are holding me back from being a powerful man of God. Is that what you want? Do you know how weak you are, Emma? You are not a strong Proverbs 31 Christian woman! Do you know what a joke you are? God is ashamed of you, allowing the devil to dry up your spirit like this! I will never get ahead in the church while you are dragging me down! You are a total embarrassment to the call on my life. You make me look bad as a man of God."

Then Alan came nearer to my face like a vulture swooping in and assessing his prey. His soft, snivelling words had a spiritual stench of their own.

"You are sick, Emma, sick in your body and your mind. You have allowed the devil to possess you. Do you understand? There is nothing left of you anymore. How can you do this to me? God wants to use me so powerfully for His kingdom around the world, and by you being selfish like this and letting the devil make you sick, I will never get to be where I want to be. You will have to answer to God for this!"

I lay there in a semi-state of consciousness.

Again, Alan used his favourite threat because he knew I genuinely loved God with all my heart.

"Because of this, Emma, you won't make it into heaven – you WILL go to HELL!"

I started to cry. I didn't want to go to hell. I loved God with all my heart. I had tried my hardest to be the best Christian wife and mother. I wanted to please God and Alan. I didn't want to be like this. How had I got to this point in my health and life?

I whispered from the depths of my heart, "I love you, God, I'm so sorry."

At that moment, the Spirit took me into a vision. I saw God's huge hands, high above me in the heavens, and God's voice audibly resounded through the ceiling, "ENOUGH IS ENOUGH." I watched as God's hands clapped together, and I heard a loud sound like crashing thunder. In reverent fear, my heart acknowledged God for his supreme authority over my life. Instantly, I felt safe, and for the first time, in a very long time, everything became incredibly obvious.

Of course! Alan was the valley of the shadow of death the Prophet had fore-warned me about, and I had to pass through it. Somehow, I had to pass through *Alan*. God had told me, FEAR NOT! I was His child, and He loved me. I knew God would get me through this, and I trusted God with all my heart.

Then came a second vision. God showed me Alan had been wearing, for a very long time, a cloak called GRACE. I saw God whisk it quickly off his shoulders.

"Are you even listening to me, Emma?" Alan came at me again. His foul stench was familiar. I know where I have sensed that horrible, vile essence before! Alan's nature was the same as the demonic entity which had tried to torment Nathan and me all those years ago when it ran up and down the hallway. Now I could see; clearly, Alan had a resident evil, living inside him, and the children and I had been living with it for these past six years! He wasn't a good Christian man. He was a fake, an impostor, and a deceiver.

How dare Alan sprout God will send me to hell! I knew I wasn't crazy and far from mental. I just needed to get away from HIM! Something started rising within me. Alan WILL NOT mistreat the children and me one more moment! I was *not* going to hell, and we were *not* going to be trapped any longer! God said ENOUGH IS ENOUGH! God was going to stop it!

I just didn't know how.

Being bed-ridden, I had no strength to leave. I knew all the promises of God He gives to His children who love Him, and I was holding onto every single one of them. Over the next few days, I grasped onto God from the tip of my little toenail in hope and waited for *something* to happen!

CHAPTER 24

My Angels of Escape

Alan begrudgingly took the children to school and forcefully fed me the eight Panadol. Apart from his outstretched arm – I never saw him. As fast as he could he was out the door.

The many years of stress and anxiety had poisoned my body, and the reoccurring breakdowns had destroyed my core strength. I lay fatigued and confined to my bed, now resembling a comfortable coffin. With my head swallowed up by a paralysing fog, I was completely debilitated. My lungs raised a slight breath keeping my existence alive – only just.

Although my body was incredibly weak, my faith in God was strong, and I continued to hold onto God, believing He *was* going to rescue me. I could feel Jesus with me, and I wasn't alone. Jesus was always faithful to His word. He never left me, and He wasn't about to forsake me.

The only prayer to God I could muster was – two words. "Help me!" I mumbled these words over and over. This prayer was all I had left.

As I lay in hopeful desperation, I saw yet another vision. Alan, myself and the children all stood in a row. A black substance coated and contaminated us and appeared to be moving. I looked closer to see what the black was. They were leeches! Yes, they were attached to us and sucking our blood. Alan's body was covered so thickly with the leeches they were dropping off him and crawling onto us. These parasites were a curse. They were evil, and they were toxic. They sucked the life energy and purpose from within our lives. And yes, Alan had ushered them in.

The vision continued. I saw God holding a burning torch with a hot orange flame. I took it and held it up to my body, hovering it over the black slugs. They screamed and hissed and let loose their grip. They fell to the ground, and I was naked. I was glad to see my skin. I checked my whole body to make sure; not one was left. I did the same for Nathan, Hannah, and Sarah. I waved it around them until they too stood there free, naked and pure. I thanked God for this vision, and I knew it was a form of deliverance.

God had begun to answer my two-word prayer.

That afternoon there was a knock on the door. I didn't know, but this knock on the door would be the beginning of my freedom. Lydia, my friend from church, had come to visit me.

Alan wasn't home, so the children let her in.

Armed with a hand-made card and home-baked delights, she was my one true friend. Lydia hadn't seen me for months, and because she couldn't get in touch with me, that had made her very worried.

Lydia was small and sassy with a mane of thick, blonde hair and bright amber eyes. She was a beautiful woman of God, with the strength and courage of a lion. I knew I could trust her. Lydia came and sat gently on the edge of my bed. Compassionately, she asked me directly.

"Em, is everything okay with you and Alan?"

I just stared at her. A dutiful Christian wife never talks negatively about her husband. Alan had repeatedly told me this for years. I wanted to be honest, but I didn't know what to say. Desperate cries screamed inside me, but I remained silent. From the tortured look in my eyes, I didn't have to say a word; Lydia knew the answer.

She gently took hold of both my hands and prayed God would bring healing to *every* part of my life. It was a beautiful prayer full of tenderness. Tears trickled down my face as God bathed me in His love. *His powerful love was going to rescue me.* I clung to this prayer, and for the first time, in a very long time, I had a glimmer of hope.

Lydia said her goodbyes with a promise she would revisit me soon.

In the meantime, the elders of the church had squashed Alan's efforts to send me to a mental home. They did suggest I go to the doctors. One of the ladies in the church took me, and I came away holding a script for antidepressants. I didn't say much to the doctor. In his professional opinion, he summed up my condition just by looking at me.

The doctor said the pills don't work straight away – but for me, they did. The sertraline gave me clarity in my mind and a strength to my core. Suddenly, for the first time in six years, I could feel things shifting in my favour.

Lydia revisited me the following week with more fervent prayers for God to set me free. By now, I had shared a few of Alan's dealings, and she was able to pray specifically. I was still confined to my bed every day, but I was getting stronger. Lydia and I giggled together pretending she was God's spy sent to me on a Holy-top-secret rescue mission.

After Lydia left, Alan unexpectedly came home. He didn't see me straight away, but after a while, he burst into the bedroom and demanded to know what was going on. *Nothing was going on – except Lydia had prayed for me*. But Alan didn't know that.

Maybe he saw the two washed cups upturned on the sink? I never did anything without Alan knowing. He knew *something* had gone on in the house while he was away, and he didn't like it.

The spirit realm though unseen – is real. It is our sixth sense. It was as though the evil in him perceived his control was slipping, and Alan knew he was losing his tight grip on me.

I spoke out, "What are you doing home?"

For me to be aware he was home was a shock to him. He replied, "Nothing that concerns you. You didn't answer me! What's been going on?"

For the first time in my life, I didn't feel intimidated by Alan. A supernatural strength was flooding into me. Diverting the conversation away from Lydia's visit, I said, "I'm starting to feel better on this medication!"

He wasn't happy about the statement. He just glared at me.

Feeling confident, I continued, "Mother has always said if I ever want to have a break, I can go and stay at the beach house. I thought while it is school holidays, I might ask her to take me there for a week or so with the children. Can I use the mobile while you are here to phone her, please?"

He questioned me, "Why do you want to go there?"

I replied honestly, "I want to clear my head, and I think the cottage is the best place for that."

He snapped back, "I don't think it's a good idea, Emma, you need to rest. You are not well, remember!"

He was not happy I had made such a request. I said again, "I think it would be good for my health!"

Alan's disposition intensified, "I can say you are not going to go, and you won't!"

I persisted, "I would like to go! I *need* to get away and get out of this bed."

Standing up to Alan made him angry. He shouted at the top of his voice, now full of rage.

"YOU ARE NOT GOING!"

As I lay still in the bed, I tried to remain calm and just breathe. Silently, I focused on God and internally cried out my two-word prayer!

"*HELP ME!*"

Alan started pacing around the bedroom. He was fuming, and I could sense a frenzied attack from him coming my way.

I knew I had to escape this man now! I felt an open heaven appear in the ceiling again. It was the same open heaven I had years ago in my bathroom when I first talked to God. The Holy Spirit poured down into me, filled me with more strength, and God took my right hand once again.

I got up out of bed as though being resurrected from my grave.

I tangibly felt in the atmosphere, angels guiding and protecting me as I walked into the children's rooms. Maybe they were the same angels that stood on my roof-top all those years ago? The same angels that celebrated in my house when the devilish entity got his marching orders?

It didn't matter. What mattered was these angelic beings were here and helping me escape. I was amazed at what was taking place. I could see and feel angels in front of me, behind me, and either side of me. I didn't have a plan. I just did whatever came naturally to me at that very moment, and the angels covered my every move. I filled a large overnight bag with some basic things for myself and the children.

Alan was furious and hot on my heels like an all-consuming dark shadow, but he didn't try and stop me or grab me in any way. The angels were giving off so much light Alan's darkness couldn't penetrate the atmosphere. I could feel an invisible bubble of protection around me, so I just kept going and focused on rounding up the children and getting out of the house.

Alan had thrown the keys to the car on the kitchen bench. I saw them as if they were calling me to pick them up. I did and said, "Come on, kids, we are going to Grandma and Grandpa's cottage for a little holiday!"

They all resounded with a *YAY*, totally unaware of what was happening.

Alan stood in front of me. His death stare was penetrating. "YOU ARE NOT GOING?"

I looked directly at him. "Yes, I am! I am going!"

I had never revolted against Alan like this ever before. He glared at me, fiercely, and his words were slow and loud.

"LISTEN… TO… ME… EMMA! YOU… ARE… NOT… GOING!"

His next statement shocked me.

"I liked you better when you were sick!"

What an insane thing to say! *He liked me better when I was sick!* All these years, what was I to him? Some sort of pawn in his twisted, depraved, power game of life? My desperation to get away from him increased even more.

Alan positioned his body in the middle of the doorframe with his arms and legs outstretched. He did not want us to get past. I sensed his rage escalating, and I was intimidated. I feared he would become violent for challenging him.

What did God say through the Prophet? FEAR NOT! I re-focused, took a deep breath of courage, and then pushed the children, one by one, through the gaps in between Alan's arms and legs. Alan still didn't move. To my amazement, he appeared transfixed to the doorframe. I shouted to the children to hurry and wait next to the car.

This scenario was unbelievable, but now it was my turn. I started to shake because the reality of what I was doing dawned on me. Then a sensation of warm hands touched my back. They were my angels behind me, sensing I needed some support and encouragement. I heard one of them whisper, "*Keep going.*"

Alan still hadn't moved. It was as though he was frozen. I squeezed myself through the gap between the doorframe and Alan's muscular body. I was finally outside. He didn't try to stop me.

I ran towards the car, petrified Alan would pursue and grab me, but again, he didn't. I glanced back at him, now released from the doorway as he slowly shuffled towards us deflated and defeated.

The children huddled around my legs as I fumbled with the keys. I couldn't find the car key! Then I saw it, stuck it in the lock, opened the doors, strapped the kids in frantically, locked their doors, jumped in the front seat, locked my door, and started the car.

Alan, now standing by the edge of the driveway, looked numb and empty.

Once more he shouted, "EMMA JANSE, YOU COME BACK HERE NOW! YOU ARE NOT GOING!"

I put the car in reverse, wound down my window and shouted back, "YES ALAN, YES I AM… GOD SAID!"

As I drove away, I looked back. There stood a man defeated at his own game. His head hung low, and his lungs appeared crumpled and void of air.

I, in turn, took a massive breath into my lungs. It felt so good. So clean, so pure, so fresh. My mind instantly started to defog for the first time in years.

I remembered in the Bible, Lot and his wife had gone to a place called Sodom and Gomorrah; a place of gross contamination and sexual debauchery. They had become trapped, and God's wrath was about to destroy the city. Through Abrahams' pleading prayers, God had mercy on them and sent angels into the city to remove them supernaturally.

I knew this had just happened to me too.

God gave Lot and his wife one command. *Don't look back or you will turn into a pillar of salt!* Lot's wife, for whatever reason, did look back and instantly turned to salt. I heard God say; *Don't you look back either!* At that moment, I knew I would never return. We had finally escaped the evil for good.

I cried with tears of joy. The suppression I felt from Alan in and over my life for all those years lifted.

For the first time in a very long time, I knew I was going to be all right. I knew the children and I would never be going back to that toxic, dark existence ever again. As my three little cherubs sat quietly, I looked at each little face displaying complete trust in me, and although they had no idea of what had just taken place, a beautiful peace surrounded us all.

I know exactly how it feels when an animal is locked up in a cage for a very long time, being beaten every day by an evil task-master. It is a horrible existence. I know exactly how it feels when the animal longs for love and justice, and then through a sheer miracle, it is released into freedom and the abuse is finally over.

It was hard for me to believe this was happening, but it was. God had answered my two-word prayer.

I WAS FREE!

The church soon discovered Alan had sexual encounters with Alisha, a young girl in the congregation. Alan and I had taken her under our wing as her family lived in the country. When I left Alan, she felt responsible for our break-up, and had gone to the head minister and elders and told them everything. Then Alisha phoned me and confessed their affair with a sincere apology.

The church called Alan in to question him about the allegations. Alan insisted Alisha and I had severe mental problems and had conspired this story together to tear down his powerful ministry. Alan said we were both possessed by the devil.

After five hours of interviews with Alisha, the head minister and elders concluded she was telling the truth. Alan now, finally, was exposed for the wolf that he was, and immediately stood down. The executive board offered Alan counselling, but he declined as he insisted there was nothing wrong with him. This uncovering with Alisha was just the beginning. Little did I know, there was more to come.

But for me now, a new life began. I had contact with my parents and friends. I had money in my purse, food in the fridge, and peace in my soul. For the first time, I was able to choose what I wore, what I ate, what I watched on television, and I was completely free in every area of my life.

Replacing my bedding was the first on my list. After Alan's illicit affair, I left all that dirty linen behind. Walking through the shopping centre by myself, I felt strange. Strange because I could choose to buy whatever I liked.

My heart fluttered as I looked at the designs. Drawn to a rose pattern set in a background of pastel pinks and greens, it was delicate and feminine. Alan had dictated black was our colour theme to decorate our house. Masculinity and darkness always filled our home. I could hear Alan's voice booming loudly in my ear; my choice was not appropriate. A hot flush of anxiety permeated throughout my body. I fought off his oppressive sound and picked up the sheet set. I felt like a naughty little girl and giggled as I opened my purse and paid for it with my own money at the checkout.

Everyone was going about their business as usual. My shopping experience was anything but usual, though I had a glimpse of hope that one day it would become my normal.

The best part of leaving Alan proved my sanity was still intact. I wasn't going crazy or mental as he consistently predicted.

Over the next few months, Alan's lifestyle exposed his can of worms. Black leeches to be exact. One by one, slimy strands of evil kept presenting itself in and around his life.

What is that expression? When you are in it, you can't see it. But it was clear and made sense now I was outside looking in. Alan had been living a double life. He wore his church mask every Sunday as the charismatic Pastor, preaching, marrying couples and praying for people and then a face full of lies, cheating, stealing and self-indulgence every other day.

The leeches also exposed Alan was having affairs with four other women as well as Alisha. That was five he was seeing, as well as being married to me. Two of the women were friends of mine, and two worked at the casino. So much for his beautiful, eloquent prayer.

Alan had a string of debts over many years. One of them was a car he had bought years ago by forging my signature, which came to light when the debt collectors knocked on my door out of the blue one day and demanded hundreds of dollars. There was nothing I could do but to pay the balance. The forged signature was such a good likeness I couldn't disprove it wasn't me.

Alan used to sit for hours trying to copy my signature with a similar scribble. He told me it was a form of endearment so he could be close to my heart, a gesture of romance, and his way of feeling one with me.

Every time the phone rang, or there was a knock on the door, nine times out of ten, it was someone chasing Alan for money he owed them. He left me with thousands of dollars to repay. He had stolen money from the church and Alisha's inheritance. Her father had been sick, and I remember Alan going to the hospital to pray for healing for him. Her father died two days later. Alan comforted her, all the way to the bank. She had given him the total sum of money to invest in their new life together. After the transfer had gone through, she never heard from him again.

I did hear on the grapevine, Alan took drugs, drank alcohol and visited prostitutes all while he was pastoring, but guess what? I did believe it!

And, he never held a marriage license! One lady tracked me down years later sharing her heartache when she found out she was not legally married.

The list of Alan's misdemeanours was endless, as many black worms kept appearing steadily out of the can – for approximately five years. Though it was painful for me to face each one, it was a reminder to be grateful this wasn't my life any longer.

I did ask Alan one time about the affairs. I was curious to see what he would say. His reply was swift and cold.

"You are ruining my day!"

I didn't care about the five other women anyway. *I was free!*

Alan had irregular visits with the children when it suited him. I feared he might try and hurt them in his nasty, obscure, unbalanced manner. I prayed the good shepherd would spare His little lambs from any harm from the wolf in sheep's clothing. When Alan had them, they never went anywhere according to the children, and there was always a different woman in the house. They always returned home unclean and full of sugar but seemingly unscathed to a much-relieved mother.

One day, out of the blue, Alan phoned me. He was frantic.

"Emma, I need your help. Please, I'm desperate!"

What on earth would Alan be so desperate for that he needed my help?

Warily, I asked, "What is happening?"

With terror in his voice, he said, "You might not believe me Em, but I think I'm demon-possessed."

My jaw dropped. Does this man honestly think I am so stupid I would believe anything that came out of his mouth? He said God had shown him! I thought for once this could be the truth.

Alan seemed genuinely despairing and of course, pleaded for my help. Knowing how to pull my heartstrings, it took all my strength to say no! He insisted I was the only person he could trust. Except I didn't trust *him*.

I suggested he go to the church and take them up on their offer for counselling. If he was genuinely serious about getting help for his evil, possessed heart, he could go back and humble himself and be accountable. The elders would be happy to care for him. Submitting himself to this process would be a sure sign he was genuine. I was not the one to help him, and I was not going to fall prey to another one of his deceptive tricks to weasel back into my life. The children and I were safe now, and he couldn't hurt us anymore. He never asked the church for help.

Alan had dual citizenship for Australia and the United States. On one of his few visits to see the children, he told them he was going to New York on a business project. Of course, with Alisha's funds. I didn't care what he schemed up anymore. My heart only cared how the children were affected by seeing him.

He promised to bring them each back a pair of high-top shoes. *How did he know what size to buy?* I suggested I draw around their feet on a piece of paper. It was at that moment when I was tracing the pen around Nathan's toes; I knew Alan would not be coming back. He had no intention of getting the shoes. Nathan was eight, Hannah was five and Sarah was one. As Alan left, he told them he loved them and said to check the letterbox every week for a postcard.

It has been 25 years since that day he left. There were no postcards, no high tops, no letters in the mail, no phone calls, no birthday cards, no money, no help, no love, no encouragement, nothing. The only thing he gave them – was abandonment.

More news came through the grapevine. I tore down Alan's ministry, and the church turned on him, so he was forced to make a new life for himself. He has nothing to do with God or the ministry anymore.

God says vengeance is mine. I had to let go of any revenge. I refused to give this man power to poison me – even through my thoughts.

Now I want to take you back to two incredible threads I have also embroidered onto my tapestry.

CHAPTER 25

The Day I met my Mother

I tried to find my birth mother when Nathan was born. I had a deep longing to connect with her after giving birth to my first child. It's common for people who are adopted after they have a baby, to want to know who their birth parents are. The yearning to see where you came from intensifies. Mine did. I contacted our local Perth adoption agency but had no luck.

Not one door opened, so I left it alone.

After Hannah was born, I felt a prompting to try again. I had become a Christian since my first attempt to find her, and I felt my search was more promising now I could pray about it. My experiences with God taught me it was His will to heal and restore every broken, damaged and missing part of my life. I also knew something about God's leading and timing, so whenever I felt deeply about something, I took it to Jesus in prayer.

The craving to find my birth mother became fierce, so I kept praying.

I knew there were four children from her womb. Call it intuition or gut feeling, I just knew.

Alan and I had moved to New South Wales with his Bible studies, and I had a strong urge to contact a local Sydney adoption agency. I looked up the Yellow Pages and found the nearest branch in our area. I phoned them and gave them the only name I had. My first birth name – Mavis Patterson. A few days later the agency called back with some good news. They had found a Mavis Patterson and gave me her current address and telephone number. My heart thumped as I took down the details. This scribbled address was a map that would lead to a treasure; my genealogy riches and family jewels, buried for many years. I thanked God. I knew it was the right time and He had now opened this door.

Mavis lived in Perth, and now we were in Sydney. How ironic! But, when the timing of God is right, everything falls into place, even when there are obstacles. My brother was getting married in two weeks, and we had already purchased tickets to fly back to Perth.

As soon as we arrived home, I nervously contacted Mavis, and she confirmed she was my grandmother. After our initial shock, we shared many emotions of love, regret, and excitement. She told me, Laurie, my birth mother, was living in Broome and would let her know I had now made contact.

In the meantime, Mavis and I made our arrangements to see each other. The day came for me to meet my grandmother. I was so nervous I felt sick. Deep within me lay a secret fear of rejection. I desperately wanted her to like me.

I rang the doorbell and waited. Within a few seconds, Mavis opened the door. Of course, she was amazed to see me standing at her doorstep. She wrapped her arms around me and gave me a huge hug.

"Finally," she said, "after all these years. We have just been waiting and waiting for this day to come. You can call me Nanna!"

I replied feeling, completely, overwhelmed with her acceptance, "So have I, Nanna, so have I."

Mavis brought out every photo album she had, and we sat for hours while I learned my history. She handed me a photograph of my mother. I could have been holding up a mirror. My mother's eyes, her hair, the way she smiled; it was me. Even though I was looking at a stranger, this woman's blood and DNA were also mine.

Tears welled up from the depths of my emotions, and I couldn't stop crying. Photo after photo, stitch by stitch, my tapestry was being decorated very quickly before my very eyes. I saw photographs of relatives with their facial features, and I sat in awe as I studied their noses, eyes, and chins. There were people in the world who looked like me. These people were my beginning and my original pattern.

All my life, I used to look at others, and if there were similarities, I would think to myself; are you my family? When people met me and said, "Oh, my goodness, have you got a sister or brother, such and such, you look exactly like them" – I couldn't help thinking – maybe I do?

Mavis embraced me with all her love that day and gave me Laurie's telephone number. The plan was I would ring her at 8.00 pm that night. I was so nervous.

My stomach churned as my fingers dialled Laurie's phone number.

"Hello," a soft voice answered.

"Hello, Laurie, it's Emma. How are you?"

"Oh, Emma, it's lovely to hear your voice. I am very well, thank you; shocked – but well!" she replied with a faint, gentle laugh.

"I know, I feel the same! Oh, my goodness, this is really, happening." I said.

We were both very nervous, and it wasn't the place to start any deep and meaningful conversations. We instinctively knew we had to keep anything like that for when we were face-to-face.

Laurie asked me a question? "Would you do one thing for me?"

"Of course, what is it?" I said, without knowing what her request would be.

I could hear a quiver in her voice as she spoke, "When we meet would you meet me at the park opposite Saint Vincent's Hospital? That was where I said my last goodbye to you, and I want it to be the same place where I say my first hello."

I heard her grief and heartache from all those years ago in her voice. "Of course, Laurie," I said tearfully. I knew our first meeting was going to be deeply emotional for both of us.

"I've booked my flight already, and I arrive tomorrow morning," Laurie continued. "Maybe the next day if you are free, we can meet?"

"Yes, of course, I am free, and that would be lovely," I responded. "I can't wait to see you."

"Oh, my darling," Laurie said, "with all my heart I have longed for this day to come."

When I shared with Mother I had found Laurie, the unexpected news took her breath away. Of course, she was happy for me. She wanted me to be complete. But I sensed my revelation was as though a giant rug had been pulled out from beneath her. As Mother spoke her well wishes for me, I heard the sound of tears in her voice. I wrapped my arms around her and said, "I may have found the woman who gave birth to me, but YOU will ALWAYS be my mother."

She paused for a minute and replied faintly, "Yes, I know, but now I have to share you. You are not *just mine* anymore."

We cried, strengthening, even more, our beautiful gift of love that we shared from the moment she held me.

The next two days were nerve-racking. I had many different scenarios floating around inside my head. I knew this meeting was going to be as emotional for Laurie as it was for me. I tried to stay calm. My stomach swirled with anticipation. All I kept thinking was; *is she going to like me?*

It was a weekday, so the park was empty. I walked past the lake and saw a lady sitting on a bench. I knew this was her. Laurie saw me coming, stood to her feet and started walking towards me. She was very tall and slim, her hair; jet black. Dressed in white jeans and a red, short-sleeved shirt covered in large, white love hearts, I knew her clothing was an implicit declaration of her love.

Like a magnet, each step pulled us closer together. Laurie held out her arms, and I fell into her embrace. Our skin touched for the very first time in our lives. She was 48, and I was 30. Laurie held me for what seemed like an eternity.

It was hard to break the moment though eventually we moved back to the bench and sat down. Laurie took hold of both my hands.

She looked straight into my eyes, and her soft voice touched my soul. "You're beautiful."

"You are beautiful too!" I replied.

"I love you," she whispered.

"I love you too!"

Every cell in my body screamed with the realisation I had come from her womb. Though we were physically cut away from each other from birth, it had not severed our soul connection. Our essence of mother and child had been brought back together in a moment. We cried and talked like long lost friends. As it unfolded, we were similar in our personality, talents and life choices.

A training of shorthand and typing led us to secretarial positions. We were both creatives and shared the same deep passion and flair for art and design. Remarkably, at the same age, we both fell pregnant to men of Scottish descent. I looked like her, and our voices had the same tone. It was truly amazing.

There was one difference. Laurie followed the New Age spiritual path and had become a practising white witch, and I had met Jesus and followed Christianity. We were both spiritual, but just like two magnets, we were poles apart.

Laurie pulled out a photograph from her jean pocket. In the picture, there were three people: my half-brother and two half-sisters. *I was right*. There were four of us from her womb, and my brother and sisters were exceptionally tall.

Laurie continued sharing. "I used to call you a name, you know, when you were growing inside me – *my little one* – and look at you now compared to your brother and sisters."

"I know," I replied, "I am the oldest and the shortest." Her prediction of my pet name turned out to be true. I was her little one, after all.

We had another long hug. As Laurie held me, our souls entwined together again. There was no time lapse between us. It was an incredible spiritual and healing moment for us both. She was my mother, and I was her child.

Laurie shared honestly and openly about my conception and her attempts at one stage, to try and commit suicide and self-abort me with a knitting needle. I couldn't believe what she was saying, but it appeared to me, she had to release her transgressions. I sensed she needed me to forgive her, and in some way, set her free from her guilt. Of course, in my heart, I did. I felt like I was in a dream, anyway! You know, one of those, 'this isn't happening to me' moments, except it is. Being completely detached from my reality, somehow it didn't upset me.

Laurie shared about staying at Aunt Gretta's house and going home for visits. She explained how Nanna concealed her under the vast white bed sheet to usher her into the house so no one would see her and her ever-growing belly. She told me how her father walked around the house in a drunken stupor shouting *what a calamity* she had brought into their lives. When I heard Laurie say the word calamity, I was stunned! That's the word Isabelle and I received the night we prayed. Laurie had got my attention now, and my ears pricked up with astute anticipation at what she might say next.

Laurie continued to tell me that her only refuge was in a musty, dark brown wardrobe in the spare room, and she had to leave it open just a crack for fresh air. Despite her strategies for safety, I always became extremely agitated inside her womb while she stood frozen with fear in her anxiety. She told me I would kick and spin frantically while inside her womb and there was nothing she could do to soothe me.

Laurie explained she rubbed her belly and spoke to me repeatedly saying, "It's all right, my little one, it's all right!"

At this point, I transitioned from unbelief to shock. Laurie did not know about my wardrobe phobia and significant anxiety issues which had plagued me my whole life. She didn't know when I was a little girl I couldn't sleep if any wardrobe doors were open – even just a crack. She didn't know, now, as an adult; I always closed the wardrobe door before I got into bed every night and still suffered from trauma because of this.

Suddenly, the impact of this phenomenon became a shocking reality. The transference of Laurie's stress and my remembrance of this traumatic event happened when I was growing inside her. I don't think I could have had a more incredible epiphany than this!

My phobia, anxiety and mental health issues started in her womb?

Now I knew the answer to my lifelong question – how and why?

As I sat next to Laurie, I could feel how easily the transference of her anxiety could pulsate through me as well. We had just had a hug outside her womb, and our essences permeated into each other. How much more then, being attached to her by an umbilical cord. I didn't know all the medical and biological explanations as to how this happens. *I just knew it did!*

I was living proof this was true. Stress, anxiety and phobias and goodness knows what else can be transferred and imparted into the unborn baby growing inside the womb, on an emotional, mental, spiritual and tangible level.

"You know Emma," Laurie said wistfully, "if I had kept you, my father, your grandfather, would have slowly crushed and destroyed your soul. He hated your very existence. For that one reason alone, I couldn't keep you."

"I understand," I reassured her.

I never said anything to her about my fear of the wardrobe door. I didn't want her to feel any more guilty than she already did.

Eventually, she married Dante and had his two children, Reece and Gemma. Laurie had married a man much like her father. Dante's aggression and abuse were heightened by vast amounts of alcohol to cope with the post-traumatic stress from his involvement in the Vietnam war. He would have flashbacks and re-enact war-torn events. One time he held a gun to Laurie's head shouting at his children to hide under the safety of the table, which in his mind, was base camp. At other times her children were the enemy, and he raged a verbal and physical war against them.

Laurie feared for their lives every day. At 14 and 15 years of age, Reece and Gemma were on a daily dose of Valium to cope with life. Laurie stated the obvious – if she had kept me, Dante would have been my stepdad. She told me quite plainly I might not have survived him, literally.

I saw the life I would have had if she had kept me, and I finally understood and was grateful I was adopted. Even though Graham had abused me, I believe I had the lesser of two evils, because I had two beautiful parents and a grandmother who loved me deeply. And for that, I was very grateful.

Laurie kept sharing her history. She left Dante and later married a second time. Mark was a lovely, gentle, man, and Laurie gave birth to her fourth child, Estelle. Peace and true love had finally found her.

Gina had extended an invitation for Laurie to come to the family home for lunch after our meeting. Laurie politely accepted. As my two mothers sipped tea and shared their stories, I sat back in awe and wonder.

Laurie thanked Gina for giving me the life she couldn't, and Gina thanked Laurie for giving her such a gift in me. Both women held their heads high above their obvious insecurities and intimidations. Though the atmosphere was both bitter and sweet for them, I had a sense of completeness.

In the years that followed, Laurie and I tried to find common threads despite the different paths we had taken.

Laurie assured me I had her psychic gift, which she had passed down to me. She was excited to train me as a medium and crystal healer and impart her witchcraft knowledge. But I had met and chosen Jesus, and I knew the Wicca religion wasn't my destiny. The Bible is clear these paths are not to weave together. In rejecting her offer, she believed I rejected her.

While we tried over the years to have a mother and daughter relationship, spiritually we clashed. Laurie became very bitter in her later years. Many a time she would write horrible letters to everyone and earned herself the nickname, poison pen. She was never able to heal the pain from her childhood, having to give me up, or the abuse from her father and first husband.

She said spells and affirmations to bring her relief, but Laurie never found freedom. I shared how much Jesus loved her and wanted to heal her spirit, soul, and body. I shared many personal victories I had received over the years.

Laurie believed in Jesus, but she wasn't going to surrender her life to Him.

If I wasn't going to leave my religion for her witchcraft, there was no way she would leave her witchcraft lifestyle for my belief.

And it was on that note our tune finished.

I also met my Aunty Lucy, Laurie's younger sister. She is only five years older than me, and we are also similar in many ways. Over the years, we have become great friends, and when people see us together, they ask if we are sisters and we laugh, and Lucy says; "Emma is my niece!".

In this world, I now knew where I had come from, and it was wonderful.

But I was only half complete.

CHAPTER 26

The Day I met my Father

Before my relationship with Laurie ended, I asked her for my father's name or anything else she knew about him that could help me find him. She rose in anger and promptly stated, "What, you want *more* rejection, do you? He didn't want to know you then, what makes you think he is going to want to know you now? I will take his name to my grave. I am *never* going to tell you."

I apologised for upsetting her and bowed out gracefully, but the desire to find my father increased.

When Aunty Lucy found out Laurie had reacted this way, she went under the family radar and with the help of some distant cousins, found the name and address of my birth father. Incredibly proud of her secret detective work, Aunty Lucy phoned me and announced his name. "Emma, your birth father is Douglas Williams!"

Well, it wasn't proven yet, but after sending Douglas a detailed personal letter and some photographs, I waited to receive the results from his DNA test. And, after weeks of suspense, it came back 99.991% positive.

Douglas lived in Perth and only 45 minutes away from me. I'm not sure if I was more nervous about meeting my mother or my father. I thought it would have been a bit easier doing it all a second time, but it wasn't.

Douglas gave me the choice of where we would meet. A park setting had been perfect with Laurie, so I suggested one near to both of us. Again, it was a weekday, and the park was empty. Douglas was already sitting on a bench when I arrived. He saw me coming and immediately stood to his feet and started to walk towards me. My heart started thumping. I broke out in a sweat, and my legs began to shake, so I took some deep breaths.

Douglas held out his arms and said, "My baby girl!"

Now, my whole body was shaking. Douglas grabbed me tightly. His embrace was warm and firm.

"And you are my dad!" I whispered as tears rolled down my cheeks.

Douglas took my face in both his hands and stared into my eyes. I looked into his, and at that moment, our souls seared together. We spoke no words. There was no need. There was no denying the essence of genetic love permeating in and all around us. This man was my father, and I was his child.

Douglas shared how lucky he was to have finally found me. He held my hands and never let them go. We talked all afternoon on that park bench. For five hours to be exact. He was happily married for 40 years to his wife Olga, and they had two children. A boy, Damien and a girl, Amanda. Another brother and sister I instantly inherited.

He shared his childhood family history, much of which was sad, dysfunctional, shocking and heartbreaking. Both my birth parents had their struggles with abuse and skeletons in the closet. After hearing from Laurie what my childhood would have been like if she had kept me, and now understanding what Douglas was telling me, I was once again very grateful to be adopted.

Douglas said, "Immediately, I knew you were mine from a photo you sent me."

I replied, "How?"

"Well, I could see your hands," he said, as he placed his palm firmly against mine. We both had crooked little fingers.

Douglas spoke proudly, "My mother, that is – your grandmother, me and you, are the only ones in the family to have bent little fingers. As soon as I saw them in one of your photos, I knew you were mine even before I had the DNA test."

As he held my hands, I had a rush of sexual attraction. What on earth is going on? The pull was so intense towards him; I had to fight it with every part of my being.

I knew he sensed my reaction, and I felt dirty and ashamed.

I had been single for eight years and had no interactions with men. I thought maybe I was craving touch and intimacy within my subconscious, but it was far more profound than that.

Douglas stared intently into my eyes with his fierce, light-blue gaze, penetrating right into the very core of my soul.

He continued to open up. He and his mother had a physically close relationship. They didn't have sex, but they used to kiss. He loved his mother deeply in this unnatural dynamic. After she died, he pined for their connection. As he sat there, he started to share his sexual desires for me.

I felt like I was on the Jerry Springer show.

Douglas had always known about me. With that knowledge, he created a fantasy relationship with me – in his mind. It started when I turned six. He had worked out my age from the year I was born.

This fantasy relationship was daily. Douglas formed innocent images of us doing things together that daddys and daughters do. Then, 12 years later, when I turned 18, the images changed. Douglas began a sexual relationship with me – in his mind. I was now 38, and for 20 years, Douglas had projected all this lustful energy towards me.

I can't describe the power and force behind the sexual pull. It smothered me like an oversized coat that I couldn't take off. Douglas also told me he was a skilled hypnotherapist and used to hypnotise his two children regularly for fun. As he stared intently into my eyes, the sexual pull became fierce, and I was sure he was trying to hypnotise me. Douglas seductively suggested our meeting might be more comfortable taken to a motel room.

Of course, I knew this was wrong. Douglas is my biological father. I am his child. A father and daughter cannot have sex together, AND…

it is a fundamental Biblical moral. It took *all* my willpower to resist his invitation.

I awkwardly said goodbye to Douglas that day, feeling trapped by his sexual advances which never left my thoughts and emotions. We had plans for more visits, and I knew I needed help to be set free from this spiritual lustful snare.

I lived in a continual state of desiring to have sex with Douglas regardless if he was with me or not. No matter how hard I tried to push the sensations away, they would not leave me alone. A generational stronghold of lust tormented me.

I shared my plight with two trustworthy Christian friends who I knew would understand and wouldn't judge me. I asked them to help me pray and break these incestual chains which had trapped me in a mental, physical and spiritual bondage.

For three months, we prayed. There was no release. Then one night, I was peeling carrots for dinner, and a vision appeared in front of me. I can only describe it as a massive pile of black excrement. I stopped what I was doing and started to pray in tongues. The mound grew larger and larger before my eyes. Two infra-red laser beams appeared from within the pile and stared at me. It was vile. Twenty years of accumulated black sexual filth from Douglas was right in front of me.

I looked straight at it and said with authority, "In the name of JESUS, I break the power of this sexual spirit upon my life, and I command you GO and leave me alone!"

As quick as a flash, it vanished! "Oh, my goodness! Did you see that God? It's gone!" I exclaimed, astounded at what was taking place. Immediately, I knew I was released. "Thank you so much, my loving Father. You care about every part of my life, and you want me to be free."

I phoned my friends straight away, and they were pleased and thankful our prayers had reached God.

The next time I saw Douglas, he still advanced his affections towards me, but they had no impact. His lust couldn't penetrate me anymore.

Over the next few months, Douglas and I spent time together getting to know each other, but it was always uncomfortable.

His love for me was all-consuming, and he couldn't control his desires. He wanted to take me to America to a County where it is legal for a father and daughter to get married. It was bizarre. Poor Olga knew of his obsession with me and had to seek counselling for her husband's affair even though it was mental and one-sided. I was the other woman, and I felt like one. It was the most sickening place to be as his daughter. If this has surprised you – imagine how surprised *I was!*

We undoubtedly shared a biological affinity, though I had to decide to stop seeing him. I was fearful of his warped influence on my children. My number one priority was to protect them.

Also, a man in the church had asked me out on a date, and Douglas was outraged with jealousy. Another reason this evil dysfunction had to stop!

I said my goodbyes to Douglas and asked him to respect my decision for no more contact. To this day he has obliged to my request.

I don't have a relationship with either of my birth parents now, but I can lay to rest my questions and deep longings of who I was. Also, I was able to break the generational curses God had shown me were in my blood-line.

I have physical and character traits which are the same as my birth parents without knowing them. There are parts of myself which are identical to my adoptive parents, as I have spent my whole life with them. In the psychology debate between nature versus nurture and which one has the most significant influence on a human being, I am proof that both are true.

CHAPTER 27

Life After Alan

You know those t-shirts people wear with the bold statement – WE SURVIVED… whatever it was – it's their declaration to the world that they conquered a seemingly impossible challenge and a task that took immense determination and courage. One they thought they could perhaps die from in the process, but they pressed on despite harrowing conditions and death-defying pain. A significant trial maybe not everyone could survive. But they did!

The tsunami didn't drown them; the prison didn't break them; the mountain didn't claim their lives.

Seriously, from the utter relief of escaping Alan's daily abuse, I wanted t-shirts made for myself and my children to wear as a reminder of how strong and victorious we had been!

We would wear the shirts with pride as a trophy of our endurance and bravery – a keepsake about a tale of survival that changed the pattern of our lives forever.

Our t-shirts would read – WE SURVIVED ALAN JANSE!

When the children and I arrived at the cottage, after obtaining our freedom, I was free, but my overall health was not good. The years of abuse had taken its toll and daily life now for me was a struggle.

I developed chronic fatigue and acute anxiety. I prayed in faith every day for healing, but my condition remained the same.

The antidepressants helped somewhat, but I knew it was just a Band-Aid, and one day I would have to deal with what was underneath – but not today. Today was only about surviving the moment.

We go through different seasons in life – Winter, Summer, Autumn, Spring, and we know winter seasons are incredibly bleak and stormy. God was allowing me to walk through some things in my life which were extremely hard.

It was tempting to think God had deserted me. But when I sat before Him, promises from the Bible washed over me declaring of His great love, protection and perfect will. I struggled to believe that my present condition could be part of His grand design for my life, but God spoke a passage in Psalm 139 verses 13 to 18 that became my anchor for this trial and gave me immense comfort.

> "For You formed my inward parts;
> You covered me in my mother's
>   womb.
> I will praise You, for I am fearfully
>   and wonderfully made;
> Marvelous are Your works,
> And that my soul knows very well.
> My frame was not hidden from You,
> When I was made in secret,
> And skillfully wrought in the lowest
>   parts of the earth.
> Your eyes saw my substance, being
>   yet unformed.
> And in Your book, they all were
>   written,
> The days fashioned for me,
> When as yet there were none of them.
> How precious also are Your thoughts
>   to me, O God!
> How great is the sum of them!
> If I should count them, they would be
>   more in number than sand;
> When I awake, I am still with You".

I looked up the Hebrew root word for wrought, and it means to embroider. God embroidered me together in Laurie's womb. I was an original, woven masterpiece. Just like an intricate tapestry. All those tiny stitches placed so perfectly. All my colours were blending purposefully with exact precision. And if God's thoughts towards me outnumbered every single grain of sand in the whole world, I had to trust the master weaver knew what He was doing.

When I left Alan, I thought the storm was over. Little did I know a heavy rain had just begun to fall. My life was harder now than it had ever been. The result was, I had to depend on God for *everything*. These debilitating health conditions were my winter season, and ahead of me was a long, cold winter, but every day I lived in a quiet, determined, faith-filled, bull-dog tenacity hoping one day I would be well.

Nathan, Hannah, Sarah and myself attended church every Sunday. The children were active in Sunday School and the Youth Group. I did my best to keep them secure and grounded.

After Alan's actions in the church had come to light, overnight, my whole life dynamic changed. I never imagined I would be a single parent with chronic health conditions, but I was. Now my full-time job was bringing up three children to the best of my ability. Three children who lived with their own suppressed issues of abuse they had incurred from their father. Years of unjust trauma and now abandonment.

My chronic fatigue and anxiety were so debilitating, I was unable to work, and I was incredibly grateful the Government granted me a disability pension.

Overwhelmed with the task set before me, I had no choice but to *accept* this was my lot in life for now. This was another challenge I was determined to succeed at with all my heart. It was my calling and my duty as a mother.

Having to bring children through the effects of trauma and abuse is no easy thing, especially when we were all broken, but with unconditional love, and strength from God, I knew – all things were possible.

My beautiful parents Ralph and Gina stepped up and helped financially, physically and emotionally. I thanked God for His great plan in orchestrating them to be my parents. In hindsight, I couldn't have endured this trial without them.

Time went by, and life was hard.

I continued to pray and ask Father God for healing. I knew the healing scriptures. God had healed me in the past. I had other prayers answered. But not this one.

God is Sovereign. I knew His ways are higher than our ways, and His thoughts are higher than our thoughts, so I just had to trust Him, even when I didn't understand the whys.

I found a scripture in my Bible. 2 Corinthians 12 verse 9, "And He said to me, My grace is sufficient for you, for My strength is made perfect in weakness. Therefore, most gladly, I will rather boast in my infirmities, that the power of Christ may rest upon me".

It was here in my weakness I cried out to God, and I found His love for me more deeply than ever before.

I began to realise my valley in Psalm 23 was not over. Submerged in the depths of hardship and illness, I leaned on Jesus for everything, and I forced myself to trust Him broken.

Scriptures I had taken for granted in the good times now shone brightly with a whole new perspective. Philippians 4 verse 4, "Rejoice, in the Lord *always!* Again, I will say Rejoice!"

I *had* to rejoice even when every part of my life and existence was full of sickness and grief.

My daily routine was heavy and hard! Kind of like pushing a parked bus up a hill, *every day!*

One hard day rolled into another and week after week, month after month, year after year, there was no relief, except the outpouring of God's love to carry me through. I found my 'Footprints in the Sand' poem, and I found great comfort from it once more.

I knew if I didn't draw my strength from the Holy Spirit, I was not going to make it. God wanted to show me the deep things of Himself, and I had to choose to abandon myself to the process.

I wanted to swim in God's clear blue sea of natural blessings. Who likes jumping in a deep, cold ocean in the black of night? Not me! But that is what I had to do. I found myself in the dark cold, uncharted waters, and I wondered why this was happening to me. I knew God would NOT let me drown, *though every day it felt like I was!*

I sat daily at the feet of Jesus in prayer, the one who said, He would never leave me nor forsake me. And, Jesus never did! I used the hardships of my lessons to build my faith and relationship with God. For that one reason alone – all the pain, grief and turmoil of life – was worth it.

I used my newfound experiences to teach my children the basic morals and values of being a decent person, and that with faith, hope and love in God – you can accomplish anything.

I taught them to be accountable for their actions, that there are consequences to their choices; good and bad – *and to always tell the truth, no matter what!* After living with Alan's compulsive lying disorder, untruths could not be a part of our lives.

Just the thought of someone lying to me made me instantly nauseous. Yes, Alan's warzone was over, but now somehow, I had to learn how to walk again on this road of life. I had to learn to step forward without the feeling of being in a minefield of fears – past, present and future – with everyone I met.

In the aftermath of Alan, I had become a nervous, timid and worn-down woman. I could somewhat relate to the war-battled soldier who had returned home. I had gained freedom, but my wounds had left me deeply scarred, and subsequently left me with PTSD; post-traumatic stress disorder, which trapped me in a mental war of thoughts and triggers.

I constantly battled thoughts of suicide, but my determination to be the best mother was more forceful in my internal dialogue. I had an incredible love for my children's innocent and vulnerable lives, and my responsibility and duty of care for them outweighed my crisis.

Every day the children posed questions starting with why, and they often asked me, "Are you going to get back with Daddy?" Where was Daddy anyway? At this point, no one knew.

They didn't know about all the illegal and unfaithful antics their daddy got up to as a church Minister, and I wasn't going to explain that to them. I could only describe it like this.

"You know my favourite pottery vase on the mantelpiece over the fireplace? That vase is Mummy. Daddy has knocked it off a few times, and it has broken in large pieces that Mummy was able to glue back together. But this last time when Daddy knocked it off, it smashed into thousands of tiny pieces, some as fine as dust. Even if Mummy wanted to try and glue it back together, it is not going to be possible. It's unfortunate, and I'm sorry I can't fix it this time – but that is just how it is. So no, Mummy and Daddy are not getting back together."

The stress I was under took its toll on my long brown hair. I awoke to find clumps of dark strands on my pillow every morning, and handfuls washed away in the shower. I lost two-thirds of my hair in one week. I had developed alopecia. I had to have my crowning glory cut very short, and now I resembled a plucked chicken with mange disease where clumps of hair fall out.

I cheered myself up by being thankful I was alive and not facing a terminal illness, although, from my appearance, it looked like I was. When I left Alan, I was 32 years old. I looked and felt like I was 100. Mother would say to me; there is always someone worse off than you. That may seem like an unsympathetic statement, but it made me focus and be grateful for what I did have.

My body crumbled away on the inside as my central nervous system broke down. Every day I got a little bit worse. It felt like I was *never* going to get better. There was NO light in sight of this seemingly very, long, dark tunnel.

I saw women being spoilt by their husbands as they complained they never had enough. Breaking a nail was the extent of their life crisis! I wanted to shake them and shout, are you CRAZY? But I couldn't. I would have looked like the crazy one!

Believe me; it was so tempting to sit around and feel sorry for every part of Emma. It was an internal fight not to. I kept reminding myself I had three significant responsibilities – my children. I loved them with an indescribable love.

What is the great mystery about maternal love? Out of nowhere, immense joy flooded me every time I held my child in my arms. As a family, we shared laughter and tears; quirky sayings evolved through our personalities, and we developed a dependence which bonded us together. Slowly the memories of our past were being replaced with happiness.

The beach cottage soon became our sanctuary. It was a place where true peace could finally reside, not just in the atmosphere of our home, but also in our hearts.

My illness raged on, hindering my ability to give my children one hundred percent of myself. I had to think of a strategy to make daily life a natural flow. God blessed me with an idea to create a family legacy. LOVE SHARE AND CARE. There was only one main rule in our house. Everything we said or did had to line up with these three words.

Is it loving; is it sharing; is it caring?

It became a part of our routine. Wash your hands before you eat, brush your teeth before you go to bed, AND… love, share and, care. Nathan was eight, Hannah was five and Sarah was one, and even though the children were small, they understood, and we soon flowed in waves of respect and understanding.

It also broke the pattern of teasing between siblings, an iron brand that had burnt me considerably in my childhood. My children were not going to be mean to each other. We loved each other, shared and cared for each other above any material want, desire or advertised necessity.

Soon our little cottage became known as the *House of Love* as anyone who came through our doors was given the same treatment. Most days held dramas and difficulties, but we tackled problems with consideration and kindness, and our little home dynamic worked in every way.

The children climbed the tall gum trees in the back yard and tied sheets from branch to branch making free-form hammocks. I made sure the knots were secure because these little monkeys would swing in their home-made nests. They stayed suspended all day reading, drawing and chatting while eating lunch and snacks I brought them.

Other days, we moved the furniture to the edge of the living room, and I sprayed Mr Sheen, a wax cleaner, on the vinyl floor. We put thick socks on our feet and pretended we were skating on ice, slipping and sliding and trying our best not to fall over. But of course, we did.

One day a lady came to visit us and slipped over on the floor. While we picked her up with great concern, she couldn't understand what had made her lose her footing. Trying not to laugh under our breath, we thought that should be the end of our skating days in case our visitors broke some bones. That would NOT be funny!

Rugs and pillows thrown over furniture made cubby houses in the lounge room, and various plays were performed with props from the dress-up box. Our house forever was filled with chatter and laughter, snuggles and cuddles, movies and pizza. There were constant play days and overnight sleep-overs, as their friends from school loved being part of the spontaneous fun and unconditional love we lived.

One child explained our home to me like this: "*I love coming to your place, Mrs Janse. When I walk through the door it always feels like your house hugs me.*"

Out of the mouth of babes!

Because of where we had come from, I was forever thankful, and I took nothing for granted. We had moved from a life of daily chaos and terror to a place we could safely lay our heads at night. There is no better feeling than that.

Ralph and Gina stayed with us often, helping me parent in my condition, which fluctuated daily. They took us on picnics and outings to the beach and bought us ice cream.

All I yearned for was a healthy, normal life.

Still depressed and exhausted, there were many days I couldn't cope. Trying to explain such things to a child was difficult, so I shared analogies.

When the children wanted my focus and energy or friends over to play, I would recite something I had once heard.

"Darling child, just imagine Mummy is a roast dinner!"

That always got a giggle.

"I'm the plate, and you are the food. First comes the meat, next, the carrots, the potato, the Brussel sprouts."

That always got a *yuck!*

"Now the cauliflower and hold on, here come the peas! And more peas, and wait, some more peas still. There are too many peas! Too many peas on Mummy's plate and they are rolling off and crashing to the ground!"

"Oh, NO!"

The children knew this was a disaster!

Then I would explain, "What you are asking right now is just too many peas for Mummy to put on her plate, and if I do, it will all come crashing down." Which in reality was a month in bed if I did too much. They seemed to understand easily, as little children do and accepted it as fact. Living in this dynamic was just how our life rolled. Whatever they wanted might be too many peas for Mummy, and that was okay.

One of my favourite things I made up was our DNA hugs. I would hug each child tightly and assure them we were swapping little particles of love.

While we were hugging, we shouted, "*GWEEZE! All my love inside you, and all your love inside me!*"

We gweezed for a long time until we were overflowing with love. The abandonment of their father had left them broken and empty, and it was my obligation to fill them up.

Restoration was happening, and though it was slow – it was steady and dependable.

One afternoon Hannah's best friend Suzie came over to play. She was one of my favourites, and we always had little chats.

Hannah was somewhere else at the time and wasn't around to hear what Suzie shared.

Suzie spoke quite straightforwardly, "Hannah's dad did nasty things to her, didn't he?"

I took a deep breath, not wanting to revisit my thoughts, and replied, "Yes, unfortunately, some people are not as nice as us!"

Suzie said, "I know, Hanny told me all about the gaffer tape!"

My stomach sank. Alan had black gaffer-tape he used for patch-ups on our black, vinyl lounge.

I braced myself and asked, "Can you tell me what Hannah said to you?"

"Well," Suzie straightened up with importance, "Hanny said when you were resting in bed, her dad asked his friend over. He would take Hanny and Nathan into Nathan's bedroom and rip a big bit of black gaffer tape off and stick it over their mouths. He did it to both of them."

I instantly felt sick. I didn't want to know anymore, but I needed to. I tried not to look shocked and calmly asked, "Did Hanny say what friend?"

"Yes, it was always Alisha from church."

I knew this was true, as Alisha visited our home regularly. I had an instant flashback. When Alisha came over, I was always incredibly annoyed, and I had to ask God to forgive my bad attitude every time. It wasn't my character to behave this way towards guests, but now I knew they had an affair, so my resentful perceptions at the time were right.

I gave Suzie a big hug. I think I needed it more than she did.

Later that evening, when Hannah and I were alone, I asked her to come and sit on my bed. My room was a safe place; a quiet place; a place of love and security. She confirmed what Suzie said was true.

"Yes Mummy, Daddy pressed the tape hard on my mouth. Then he did the same to Nathan."

I asked quietly, "What did Daddy do then?"

Hannah hesitated, then said, "He tipped up the Lego bucket onto the floor and told us to sit still and play, and not come out for any reason, big or small. We were not allowed to disturb him and Alisha."

"How often did Daddy do this to you?" I enquired.

Hannah replied, "Lots of times."

I had to ask. "Did you know what Daddy and Alisha were doing?"

"Well, sometimes they were in the pool, laughing, giggling and splashing. And sometimes, if you were at the church, they came inside the house, and I think they were doing exercises."

I nodded rapidly, "Oh, yes, probably." I saw the real picture, but I'm glad she didn't.

Hannah continued, "But Daddy taped our mouths shut too when you were resting in bed, and he was just watching television. He said we were annoying and had to leave him alone."

The thought of my children sitting for hours in Nathan's room, alone and stifled with gaffer tape stuck over their mouths made me furious.

"What if you wanted a drink or the toilet?" I asked.

"No, Daddy said we had to stay in our rooms until he said we could come out! Nathan and I talked to each other with our eyes. If I wanted to swap a bit of my Lego with him, I would hold up my piece, look at his Lego block and then he gave it to me. I used my manners. I said thank you with my eyes."

My heart broke.

"I'm so sorry Daddy did that to you both!"

I held my beautiful child in my arms and poured as much love into her as I could. Hannah shared her child-like perception.

"Daddy was mean and naughty. He should have been swimming with you, not Alisha."

I held back my tears. "Yes, my darling, Daddy should have."

As young as she was, she knew what was right and what was wrong. Hannah kept sharing, and my heart kept breaking. It was as though she was released now to speak, and she had to tell all.

"Then Mummy, after hours of us sitting there, Daddy would come back in and rip the tape off quickly. He smiled as if it was funny and said, *this is going to hurt*, and it did. When he left the room, I ran and looked in Nathan's bin to see if my lips were stuck to the tape, because every time it always felt like Daddy had ripped my lips off."

I took her face gently in my hands. "Why didn't you ever say anything to me?"

Hannah hesitated again.

"It's okay," I said reassuringly, "you can tell me."

She stuttered, "Well... Daddy said if we ever told you he would kill us."

She sobbed in my arms and released the years of this suppressed secret. I gently rubbed her back with my hand. She looked up at me as the tears ran down her cheeks and said, "Daddy never said I couldn't tell Suzie. Did I do the wrong thing, Mummy?"

I held her tightly.

"No, my darling, you have done the right thing by telling me. Daddy won't kill you. I won't let him! I love you so much, and I won't let him hurt you ever again."

I was fuming. Here I was, trying my best to forgive Alan, and now if possible, I despised him even more. I wouldn't put anything past him. I had to ask her there and then.

"Hannah, did Daddy ever touch you here?"

I placed my hand in between my legs. Hannah shook her head, and I believed her and thanked God. I didn't care how many women he fooled around with, the fact he didn't interfere with the children was a blessing! I knew God had protected my children from this man.

I talked to Nathan that night to air the hidden secret. He confirmed everything Hannah had said, and I comforted him as well. Now it was all out in the open; I thought the impact of this on their lives might go away. But Nathan was angry and plotting a way to kill his father.

Nathan burst into my bedroom one morning and stated, "I have worked out the best plan!"

"The best plan for what?" I asked.

"The best plan to kill Daddy!" Nathan replied.

I sat up, stunned at what he had just said.

Nathan proceeded to tell me, confident in his strategy. "I'm going to buy a big, long coat and get a shotgun! I'm going to catch a plane to wherever Daddy is – I'm going to find him – and then get my gun out and shoot him!"

I couldn't believe this once gentle, loving little boy would ever think up anything like this, and more to the point, he shouldn't have to. They say the age of seven is the worst age for a father and his son to be separated – even without any trauma. To see Nathan's life riddled with inner turmoil at only eight years of age was heartbreaking.

Nathan's teacher told me, every recess, Nathan would sit in the corner of the basketball court and hug his teddy bear. Nathan never played or talked to anyone; just sat, looking sad, hugging the stuffed toy. I had no idea Nathan took his teddy to school. He must have smuggled it in his bag, and this bear was security and comfort. I felt helpless to Nathan's deep wounds.

A year had passed since Alan's trip to America, and there was still no contact from him. His disappearance terrified the children.

Hannah developed a stinging tummy. She wouldn't go to school, and worked herself up every morning, crying and panicking that her daddy might be in jail or dead. I didn't know where he was, but I had to reassure her that he was all right. Her episodes of stress and stomach pains continued for two years.

The doctors could never find anything wrong with her stomach. Eventually, the anxiousness and stress developed into Crohn's disease, an autoimmune disorder, which nearly took her life three times. A standard iron level is between seven and fourteen, and her iron level was one. Because it was so low, the doctors said she could have a heart attack in her sleep.

The medical diagnosis was her illness could have erupted from a childhood trauma. In her late teens Hannah had a major operation, and 36 staples later, she had three-quarters of her bowel removed. Thankfully, she didn't need a colostomy bag as the odds were 50/50 of needing one. The procedure was successful, and after a few years of remission, now she can live a healthy life, with yearly check-ups and daily medication.

The children eventually heard Alan was alive and well, but his abandonment ran deep. Nathan, Hannah, and Sarah, all at different times, broke down and blamed themselves for their daddy's absence.

As Nathan grew, so did his anger. When he turned 14, Nathan hated his dad with a deadly vengeance. Living through his adolescence was a nightmare for us all. He got in with the wrong crowd which led him into a dark time and place. Seeping through Nathan's explosive rebellion was the backlash of what his father had done to him.

Nathan smashed doors, walls, furniture, and ornaments in our little house of love. With every drunk and drug-fuelled fist of fury, he would say; *this one is for my dad*. His explosions manifested for years, as he tried to lash out at the injustice of his father's abuse.

Nowadays, I would seek counselling for each one of my children, but 20 years ago, we didn't do that.

Someone told me once; our adolescent boys are like bucking broncos. We must do our best to ride them, and just hang on until they stop kicking. I held on in prayer, frantic hope and unconditional love for 12 years until Nathan's bucking finally stopped.

There is another thread to my tapestry I regretfully have to weave in here. Thankfully it is only a small strand.

The church was very keen to see my children cared for and me married again. Timid and terrified, I hadn't dated for eight years and was still nervous around men.

A lovely elderly couple in the church took a shine to me. Robert, their son, used to be very involved in ministry. He was recently divorced. Robert had four children, but when his marriage fell apart, he left the church and hadn't attended for years.

Because of my gentle, caring nature, they thought I would be perfect for their wayward son. So, their matchmaking began.

At first introduction, I thought Robert was rude and abrupt, but I was encouraged by people in the church to date him, if not for me, they stated, as a father to my children. They persuaded me to believe since I had come out of abuse, I was judging him too harshly.

Many put forward reasons why I should marry him – the usual; I needed a man to provide and protect my children and me. I needed to have a companion and partner to explore the world with, and never be lonely. I deserved to have someone spoil me, love me, treat me like a princess – all the cliché expressions. And to be honest, a deep part of me still desperately craved love, so that was my weakness.

Robert pulled out all the stops to woo me. Flowers, chocolates, humour, kindness, understanding, love for myself and my children. Yes, Robert swept my feet right off that floor. So, against my gut feelings, three months later, I married him.

Straight after the ring slipped on my finger, Robert changed. He turned into Dr Jekyll and Mr Hyde. His past; his personality and character were not unlike Alan's, and soon an affair, abandonment of his children, and lies were revealed. Robert started binge drinking and became abusive. He dominated, neglected and mistreated my children and me, abusing us with violence, emotional blackmail, mind games, and anger. He came into our little house of love and destroyed its beautiful presence and everyone in it.

What had I done? How had I fallen down the same hole again?

The children and I endured ten months of abuse until finally, we escaped Robert. I went to the police to enquire about a restraining order. Robert found out and was furious. He exploded and walked out. The pattern from abuse to freedom had touched my life once again.

Despite everything my children have endured, now they are adults, and I am proud of them all.

Nathan married a beautiful girl, and they have children. A boy and two girls. Life has given Nathan four gifts, where he can now channel love instead of anger.

Often Nathan says, "There is no way I am going to treat my children the way my dad treated me!" I know the real depth and extent of his passion, and pride fills me for the man and father he has become.

Hannah has fully recovered and is in remission. She is a very talented hairdresser and has recently met the love of her life, and they plan to get married.

Sarah was one year old when Alan left and can't remember him at all. Growing up without a father affected her greatly. Her abandonment issues were very severe, and it has taken many years and layers for her to find healing.

She has acquired a depth well beyond her years through her cathartic journey. Sarah is very creative and musical. Using her natural talents, she hand weaves beautiful baskets and face paints. She also loves drawing, singing and writing songs.

I know God has His loving hand on their lives, and the bond we all share between us as a family is unbreakable. The unfailing hero to our formula of success – LOVE, SHARE, and CARE!

Alan eventually tried to reach out to the children – about 20 years after he had left – but it was too late. Nathan, Hannah or Sarah didn't want anything to do with him. Sadly, the sting of the song, Cat's in the Cradle, had come to pass.

CHAPTER 28

Cries from Hell

I stood in the kitchen, looking at a sink full of dirty dishes. I pulled on my rubber gloves and plunged my hands deep into the hot water and bubbles of detergent. Washing up was such a menial task; my mind began to wander. I reflected on my life and what I had come through.

I was grateful for so many things, but mainly for knowing how much God loves me and how Jesus never leaves me during my trials. Why me? I felt so privileged.

As I thought about the goodness of God, I felt the Holy Spirit surround me with a peaceful presence that became all-consuming. Lost in this beautiful moment, I raised my arms to my Lord, dripping gloves and all, in surrender and complete adoration.

Completely overwhelmed, I knelt on the kitchen floor, closed my eyes and bowed my head.

The floor became incredibly hot like fire. I realised that I was no longer just on the kitchen floor. Somehow, I had transported to another dimension. I was suspended over a darkness, looking down into a night that never ended. It was darker than black if that could even be possible. There was an eeriness swirling in the atmosphere.

I smelt a stench similar to a stagnant pond that had been rotting for thousands of years. As I breathed in the hot toxic smell, it not only burned my nostrils but coated my tongue and my taste buds. The vile flavour made me so nauseous I wanted to vomit. The smelly atmospheric substance was so thick I started choking and could hardly manage to take in a breath of air.

Suddenly, the hairs on my whole body prickled up as a sensation of fear rushed at me. *I knew what realm this was!* I had encountered this evil before. It was the same demonic essence that rushed at me up and down the passageway in my house all those years ago.

As I knelt, I heard the faint cries of distress. Cries of inescapable fear. Wails from a never-ending suffering. People were screaming out for help. The hot vile stench got stronger. It was apparent the smell was the burning flesh of these trapped ones. Skin; being burnt alive, but they never died, just burned for all eternity.

The painful sound was continuous. Their screams got louder. For them, there was no escape; no freedom; no getting out from this place; just agony and eternal torture.

I knew these were cries from hell.

God never took me any closer. All I could hear were desperate cries and piercing screams from these tormented souls.

I started to sob deeply. My heart was breaking. I was sorry these people's souls were in such a tormented, painful and tortured place. I felt so helpless. For them, it was too late to escape this foul abyss.

I have heard people say hell isn't real, or it's just one big party. If this tiny, distant glimpse of hell is any indication of what it might be like for all eternity, there is no way I would ever want to go there!

CHAPTER 29

I will Find my Way

It was now ten years since I escaped Alan, and I was travelling along okay. My damaged central nervous system, chronic fatigue, and acute anxiety were still part of my daily life.

During these hard years, I learnt to wear a smile and managed life around the outbreaks. I tailor-made days around naps and apologised for many declined invitations. Only those close to me knew the severity of my illness. I reached a point where I had to be grateful for what I had, and just – get on with it.

In my quiet times, I felt a strong impression I was going to go to America. One Sunday at church straight after the sermon, Lisa, the Pastor's wife, approached me and said God had told her to invite me to a conference in Arizona with Dr Linda Mirrett from New Creation/Life Ministries. As you can guess, I was extremely excited. Embarking on this journey with my health condition would be a challenge, but I knew God wanted me to go. With high expectations, Lisa and I set off for a teaching, learning and exciting adventure.

During one of the lessons, Dr Linda spoke on *spiritual rape*. I had never heard of this before. She explained that spiritual rape occurs when a person uses the Bible scriptures out of context either in ignorance or worse, out of purposeful lust or gain. In doing so, they harshly and unfairly violate another person. It is equivalent to rape. It is not physical; it is spiritual.

As we listened and learned, Dr Linda's team acted out a play where spiritual rape was evident. The first scene started with a lady being physically abused at home by her husband, and she phoned the Pastor for help.

She acted convincingly, "Help me, please, my husband is angry all the time and takes it out on me. He hits me, and I need help to escape. I am desperate. Can you please help me!"

The Pastor picked up his Bible and flicked through the pages, and finding a scripture started reading, "Hebrews 5 verse 8, 'though He was a Son, yet He learned obedience by the things which He suffered'. There you go; Jesus had to learn obedience through suffering. Maybe there is something you need to learn in your suffering?"

It was apparent this scripture was out of context for her given situation, and only added more abuse to her case.

The play continued. Through tears and desperation, the lady pleaded with the Pastor for help.

"But I'm bruised and hurting!" The Pastor licked his finger and flicked through more pages and spoke calmly, "Listen to this dear. In Isaiah 53 verse 5, 'but He was wounded for our transgressions, He was bruised for our iniquities: the chastisement for our peace was upon Him, and by His stripes, we are healed'. We are to be like Jesus, and your bruises are like His. Be encouraged!"

While the play portrayed an extreme example; we got the picture of how easy it is to fling scriptures around that are totally out of context. In effect, this brutal spiritual violation rapes a person's spirit. It is wrong, hurtful and disgusting.

Then it dawned on me. Alan had done this to me thousands of times. He had raped my spirit daily. The Holy Spirit fell on me in the conference room, and I started to cry. I excused myself from the session and found the bathroom. I crumbled to the floor and sobbed. As I sat there, God healed my damaged and raped spirit, soul, and mind from the years and layers of Alan using scriptures harshly at the children and me to suit his warped agenda.

Some students showed concern for my wellbeing and stood up to find me, but Dr Linda made it clear to leave me alone with God. As my wails echoed throughout the building, penetrating people's hearts, Dr Linda declared with deep sincerity to the class, "May God deal with the person who inflicted this much damage on her."

As others heard my weeping, they too started crying. Men and women suddenly realised in their walk with God, they had either been on the giving or receiving end of using out of context scriptures, or both. The damage they caused or the wounds that were exposed were now all out in the open. The whole lesson turned into a healing session for everyone.

God had brought me all this way to America to perform a deep inner healing restoration; He knew I needed it.

I developed a strong compassion for others going through similar journeys of trauma. I decided to do a home studies Diploma in Counselling with A.I.P.C. (Australian Institute of Professional Counsellors). As a full-time single mum managing my illness, doing things from home was all I could handle. I completed 22 units over two years. An achievement of which I am thankful.

It is one thing to have personal experience of abuse and another to learn about it and gain the merits of certificates. Coupled together, it becomes a powerful thing. Knowledge and experience bring wisdom and with that comes freedom and healing. At times, I was grateful for what I had been through and as strange as it may sound, counted it as a privilege.

For Hannah's rehabilitation and recovery for her Crohn's illness, we did bead craft at home, and the pearls, gems, and wire we used for her therapy unexpectedly turned into a little hobby outlet for me.

Sarah did some modelling in her teen years, and one catwalk event I got pulled up onto the stage to fill in for someone in the mature model parade. I loved doing it alongside Sarah, so I joined the adult's class.

We strutted our stuff together for five years in many community events and women's expos, which brought more healing to my self-esteem.

Looking back, Andrew had wanted me to do this when I was 20, when I had zero confidence.

Now, not being fat at 40, but modelling at 50, I couldn't help feeling I had achieved something unexpected and remarkable. And yes, I did have those thoughts – *if Andrew could see me now!*

Life's design was ingeniously giving me opportunities to confront and conquer my demons that had put me down over my lifetime. Having opportunities to be bold and confident, pushing through the tormenting voices and stepping out of my comfort zone brought natural healing. It was a lesson that whatever hardships life throws, no one is ever too old, and nothing is ever too late for victory!

Twenty years had passed since Alan had gone, and I recognised I still had niggling triggers when things were said and done to the children or myself, and I was frustrated because of it. I was aware of the dangers of negative emotions that had never been dealt with, and there was no way I wanted to grow into a bitter older woman.

Wikipedia defines forgiveness as, 'the intentional and voluntary process by which a victim undergoes a change in feelings and attitudes regarding an offence, lets go of negative emotions such as vengefulness, with an increased ability to wish the offender well.'

I thought, how on earth am I ever going to get to that place – with an increased ability to wish the offender well? For the past 20 years, some incident always arose to stir up anger in me for Alan's damage to us all. I would work so hard at releasing my negative energy and finally succeed in my heart, only to turn around and face yet another exposed violation.

I know the Bible is very clear about forgiveness. I read in Ephesians 4 verse 32, "and be kind to one another, tender-hearted, forgiving one another, even as God in Christ forgave you".

And also, Matthew 6 verse 14-15, "for if you forgive men their trespasses, your Heavenly Father will also forgive you. But if you do not forgive men their trespasses, neither will your Father forgive your trespasses".

Such a commandment is definite. I didn't want God not to forgive me of my sin. Forgiveness was my mission. To get to the place in my heart where I had forgiven Alan to the point where I could genuinely and humbly wish him well.

I had spent years praying, and like a stinging onion, I had worked hard at peeling away my resentment and loathing I had for that man. Holding anger in my heart even for one person was too many. And I wanted the subconscious violated memories gone.

Like most things in life, it is always our choice. Deciding to forgive Alan was easy. Doing it was the challenge.

God helped me once again and gave me a vision of Alan being His child. Jesus died for Alan too, and the love God had for him was so strong. Then God showed me that when I hold hate and bitterness in my heart towards Alan, it hurts Him. I didn't want to hurt God. That made forgiveness easy. I released all my anger, resentment and negative emotions because I loved God. I was finally free of all bitterness. Now when I thought of Alan, there was a softness, and I could genuinely pray for him to be blessed.

Even though I had forgiven Alan, I still felt damage inside me. I knew my valley was not quite over. I continued to pray and asked God to show me where else I needed victory for myself and the children. Seeking wholeness is our desire and finding it is the journey. No matter how long it took, I was determined to be free.

CHAPTER 30

The Loss of a Loved One

Mother and Dad organised a three-week holiday. One of total relaxation with no phones or electronic devices. It was part of my father's recovery as he had recently had a skin lesion examined. When they arrived home and checked their telephone messages, they discovered one was from the hospital. The results had come back, and Dad's lesion was a skin cancer and the most dangerous one. A melanoma.

Three weeks had passed since the urgent message, and in that time, the aggressive cancer had spread to my father's lymph glands. In the short space of 21 days, it was now too late. The doctor's report showed it was only a matter of time.

At 78 years of age, Dad began chemotherapy. His body rejected the treatment, and after one dose, he was close to death, so he wasn't able to have anymore. The doctor gave my father six months to live, though miraculously Dad held on for another 18 months.

Over that time, sharing memories, I discovered many surprising things. One of them was my father and his mother, Pearl, my grandmother – had a favourite Psalm. Psalm 23. Of course, it thrilled my heart that we all had this in common.

A few months before my father passed away, our whole family spent his 80th birthday gathered around the hospital bed with a bunch of blue balloons and one giant silver helium balloon in the shape of an eight and a zero.

In a loving chorus, we sang happy birthday, knowing it would be the last time Dad would blow out the candles on his cake. Dad knew it too. We all held back our tears as best we could and focused on our cherished memories with this intelligent, strong, wise, peaceful and respected man who was loved by all his family and adored by his little Petal.

Mother nursed Dad at home until he passed away. To witness her love and devotion was a beautiful testimony to their happy 55 years of marriage. They certainly had an incredible bliss-filled union right to the very end.

The day before my father died, Mother, Hannah, Sarah and myself gathered around his bed at home. Dad, at this stage, was unconscious from all the heavy drugs. We hadn't been able to communicate with him for over a week. We talked about our favourite moments we had shared over the years and told him how much we loved him, though he couldn't respond.

As Dad lay heavy on the bed, I read Psalm 23 as a prayer over his life, and the most astonishing thing happened. While I spoke God's beautiful words of promise, Dad's whole countenance changed, and his breathing went from a laboured heavy inhale and exhale, to a peaceful light breath. We all stood watching, amazed and emotional. It was undeniable something was happening within him when I was reading, though we will never know.

Mother was touched beyond words, as Dad had been asking her if she thought there was a place for him in heaven.

I felt inside my heart; God was preparing Dad for the last line in Psalm 23.

'…surely goodness and mercy shall follow me all the days of my life, and I will dwell in the house of the Lord forever.'

CHAPTER 31

Wardrobe Door – You are Defeated

I made a bold decision to get to the root of my life-long anxiety. To do that I knew I had to come off my antidepressant medication and see what was underneath the Band-Aid. I had been dependent on it for 20 years, so coming off was a big thing for me to attempt.

I had no idea what or how deep my emotional wound was, but I know; all things are possible with God, and for that reason, I had faith.

God opened a door for me to attend a wellness centre that helps people with depression, anxiety, and other mental health issues. I became involved in a 12-month Pathways to Recovery program. I learnt practical strategies and tools to deal with depression and anxiety.

We practised breathing techniques and studied how we can retrain our thoughts. We gathered together in group sessions and shared our brokenness. It was a safe place to recover from abuse.

One of our applications for healing was colour therapy. We were encouraged to draw positive affirmations and colour them in. As you colour and focus, saying only those words over and over in your mind, chemically something happens. The negative cells in the brain eventually are replaced by positive ones. It's called cognitive resetting.

I had learnt about this in my counselling units.

Something started to surface with all my artwork. I had PTSD towards men. As part of my healing process, I was encouraged to start dating again. Just the thought of it gave me instant anxiety.

I had shut this door very tightly, but I was willing to work with the programme and see myself worthy of attracting a kind and loving man.

Being open, at least talking to a man, was the first step in removing the Band-Aid.

I put a relationship affirmation to colour, and after a few weeks, Simon came across my path. He was kind and caring, but sure enough, the thought of dating him invoked acute anxiety. My trigger was exposed, which forced me to face my fears head-on.

I couldn't escape this immense fear of men which internally gripped me. Merely the thought of Simon phoning triggered anxiety episodes that wanted to suck me down into a black vortex of doom. I couldn't eat or sleep and spent most of my days on the toilet.

I used all my breathing techniques, scriptures, and mental strength to break free, but my anxiety only increased. I hadn't experienced these symptoms since my days with Alan.

Day and night, awake or asleep, anxiety pulsed through my body and my subconscious.

Twice the panic attacks were so bad; I phoned Lifeline, and they talked me through them.

I knew God was with me, holding my right hand, and I knew that He was allowing this to happen, so again, although I didn't understand, amidst the chaos – I chose to trust Him.

When faced with something causing anxiety, there are three options – fight, flight or freeze. The thought of having dinner with Simon sent my mind and body into a panic. I had to flee!

I told Simon I couldn't see him anymore. And guess what? The anxiety went away. But he persisted in wanting to take me out.

I faced a real dilemma. I could be a single woman for the rest of my life or confront my fear of men and force myself to work through it. I desperately wanted to be free!

I had years of experience managing anxiety and panic attacks, but I had never encountered such a stronghold like this arising within me before. I had been off my medication for six months, and the Band-Aid was off. My emotional and psychological wound was deep. I knew fleeing would not bring any healing. I had to be free from this inner turmoil which had ruled me all my life, even from early childhood. I knew that what was ahead of me was going to be one of the most significant challenges I was ever going to have to face in my life. I had to push through and fight.

Again, I prayed to God, my two-word prayer, 'help me' and waited for something to happen.

My darling mother was with me for a short stay. She just so happened to be looking at a programme on television about the study of phobias and anxieties and called me in to watch it.

They showed a young woman who had a phobia of birds. She had this disorder all her life, and it was so extreme it was classed as a medical condition. They brought in a huge eagle, and although it was a great distance away from her, it instantly triggered an anxiety attack.

She was shaking and crying, and she couldn't breathe.

Then they took her behind the scenes with a psychologist, and after 20 minutes of cognitive therapy, she came back on stage and touched the eagle with little to no symptoms. I saw her and thought, that's a miracle. If she can do it, so can I. I continued to pray for my release.

A few days later, my girlfriend Amber and I were having coffee. I was a mess. In between mouthfuls of carrot cake, I squirted my calming drops. Then I would run to the toilet. Tonight was the night Simon would take me out for dinner. Just the thought of it catapulted my mind into a negative frenzy and my body into a shaking mess. Amber, bless her heart, was trying to understand what was going on inside of me so she could try and help me.

She said, "Emma, please share what's happening to you."

I replied, "Amber, I can only explain it like this. Thoughts of fear and unknown dread swirl around in my mind. They cause a rush of adrenalin to pulsate through my central nervous system. It is so strong it feels like every cell in my body is screaming in pain. Next, raging hot injections of nausea flood over me. It feels like I am drowning in the depths of a deep, dark ocean, but I am still breathing. My internal thoughts of panic are obsessive and compulsive, and I am trapped. There is no logic in them at all. They take on a force of their own, and I can't shut them down. I can't press the off button because there isn't one. I can't stop continually thinking about dread and fear-based thoughts."

Amber asked me, "What are you afraid of Em?"

I replied, "Nothing – everything. I don't even know what sets me off. Anxiety is just there constantly in my mind and body. I can't get rid of it. I fear the past happening again; I fear the present with every breath; I fear the future of the unknown. It's like I have to, right at this very moment, sit an exam I haven't studied for, and if I don't pass it, I will die. That's the intensity."

Amber sympathised with me. "I'm sorry Em, I wish there was something I could do. You poor thing. It must be horrible?"

"It's okay Amber," I proudly perked up in my victory lane of survival mode, "I have conquered many fears in my life – Graham, anorexia, Alan and of course my phobia of the wardrobe door, so I am determined to conquer this too!"

Amber knew about my wardrobe door episodes and curiously inquired, "How did you conquer the fear of your wardrobe door?"

Without thinking about my answer, I replied, "Well, I just shut the door every night before I go to bed, and the fear goes away."

Amber paused for a second and then responded quite simply, "*That's not conquering it Em! To conquer it, you have to sleep with the doors open!*"

Her words stunned me, and in a split second, I had an intuitive insight into the reality of the wardrobe door being the foundation of my fears throughout my life right from the time I was forming in Laurie's womb.

Of course! I always shut the wardrobe doors every night. Once I closed them, the fear was gone. Then it dawned on me. I had done that to every fearful situation all my life, thinking they were out of sight, out of mind, but that didn't make them go away. I had only suppressed them and shut them out.

Instantly I felt sick. Confronting my phobia of the wardrobe door was my eagle. It all made sense. *I had to face my fear tonight and sleep with the wardrobe doors open!*

The afternoon was nearly over, and night was approaching. I cancelled dinner with Simon. There was no way I could eat anything anyway. I focused only on one thing. *I must sleep with the wardrobe doors open.* The thought of this made me hyperventilate. I had a headache and was nauseous.

Amber came to my house and talked me through strategies and prepped me for the challenge ahead. She quizzed me on what I thought would help. I felt to read Psalm 23 and place my Bible on my bedside table open at this Psalm. I prayed angels would protect me all night and surround my bed. A peace descended. The Holy Spirit was with me.

I had a strong urge to take my nail polish off and all my jewellery. I had a shower. I didn't know why I just felt I had to. It was as though I was preparing myself for something, and I needed to be pure and untainted. I felt I needed to sleep naked – just me, untouched and uncontaminated by this world and realm. Amber supported whatever I suggested.

I desperately wanted her to stay, but she declined. Amber knew this was my destiny, and I had to stand alone. She hugged me and told me to phone her anytime throughout the night if I needed her for anything. I waved goodbye to Amber and came inside. Now, the moment had come.

I walked back into my bedroom and stood in front of the closed doors. Nausea enveloped me. Taking a deep breath with my eyes shut, I pulled both the doors of my wardrobe wide open. The sound of air gushing forward was loud and chilling. It had a dark personality all of its own. I opened my eyes.

Instantly my phobia activated. A sensation of stale fog hit me, and the stench of evil penetrated my nostrils. I had never encountered anything so horrific. I froze with fear at the blackness and dread that was desperate to capture me. It was only clothes hanging up in a wardrobe, but a dark, very tangible essence swirled around in front of me. I cried out in prayer, "Jesus, help me do this!"

I stumbled backwards. With all my being, I wanted to shut the doors. The room was closing in on me. I knew I had to do this. I knew I had to go to sleep with the doors wide open. I had to push through this all-consuming reality of the wardrobe being a vicious abyss just wanting one thing; to suck me down to the pit of hell.

That was the intensity of the horrific fear I was feeling. I was very aware that this was the same sensation I felt when I was a child tucked up in my bed all those years ago.

I laid down on the bed, and curled myself up, facing the open doors. I focused, "Emma, you can do this, and everything is okay. Thank you, God. You are in this, and I trust You."

I breathed in and out slowly. I was able to calm myself a little. I was too scared to close my eyes, but gradually, I was able to and for a bit longer at each attempt. By now, it was dark, which added to my torment, and I knew I had to roll over and put my back to this black whirlpool of evil. I didn't want to, but this was the only way to push through and be free. I rolled over slowly. Nothing prepared me for what I felt next.

Surrounded by natural darkness, I could feel the blackness in the wardrobe pulling at my body wanting to suck me back into it. Another panic episode swamped me. Centring my mind, I took slow deep breaths and focused on Jesus.

Instantly, I transitioned to a meditative state. I saw Laurie in the wardrobe just like she told me. I saw myself as a tiny foetus inside her womb while she stood frozen in the wardrobe. Her father was stumbling around the house in his angry drunken stupor shouting what a calamity she had brought upon the family.

I saw myself growing inside her as a baby, buoyant in the warm amniotic fluid that surrounded me. Its substance was tangible, thick and comforting.

Her father continued shouting and stomping around the house, trying to find her. Laurie was shaking in the wardrobe with intense fear. I was trembling with anxiety inside her. As Laurie became more anxious, the amniotic fluid grew colder, causing my delicate skin to wither, and my bones to become as cold as ice. I was shaking uncontrollably inside her womb.

As I lay in my bed, watching this, I became aware I was ice cold and shaking. Somehow mentally and spiritually, I had gone back in time to this exact moment.

I didn't know what to do, except pray. I prayed to God for His love, joy, warmth, and healing to come into the amniotic fluid and penetrate right through the baby's life and restore its mind, heal its body and bring it peace. I visualised a strong barrier of protection around the baby from the fear which was trying to pulsate into its tiny soul.

I concentrated on this happening to me in this present moment of terror, as it was happening to this baby, way back then. Unintentionally, I was cognitively swapping the thought patterns in my mind right at the root cause and exchanging fear for peace, anxiety for calm.

I don't know how long I was in this state, but it felt like hours. Faces of men who had hurt me over my life appeared in front of me. One by one, I forgave them and felt a peace and release with each one.

I returned to my vision. Laurie's father was still angry and shouting. Laurie was anxious in the wardrobe. But amid all this traumatic energy, the baby was finally peaceful in her womb.

I had won the fight and claimed my victory!

As I lay in bed, I was utterly relaxed without fear, turmoil or anxiety, and I fell asleep.

In the morning, when I awoke, the wardrobe doors were still open wide. I had survived the night. I had confronted the dark, evil fear which had entered me while I was a foetus and then had plagued me all my life. I sat up and felt different because the enormous burden had lifted from my body. I was calm in my mind. I was peaceful in my soul.

I had no anxiety pulsating through me even though the wardrobe doors were left wide open. The fear in my mind which had been ingrained into me while I was in Laurie's womb 52 years ago had gone.

WOW! How incredible, exciting and phenomenal! I had broken free of the mental trappings that inhabited my subconscious mind. No more phobia. No more fear. I was finally free.

What an incredible discovery! I can't begin to tell you how exciting it was to recognise that a mother can pass on trauma and mental health issues to her unborn child. I would never have thought this was even a possibility. Now, I knew I was living proof it was a reality.

In hindsight, finding my birth mother was not only for my healing journey but to prove that womb trauma is a reality and does exist.

There was no way I could have known about Laurie hiding in the wardrobe and passing her anxieties into me. I was adopted.

I had also just proven cognitive therapy works at a deep mental and spiritual level, regardless of your age, even going as far back as before birth.

What an important message for all expecting mothers. I had no understanding of this from a medical perspective, so I decided to research the transfer of anxiety from a mother to her unborn baby.

I was astounded as I read many biological facts at what I discovered.

Mothers who are stressed in pregnancy transmit stress to their unborn baby as early as 17 weeks.

It all has to do with the stress hormone cortisol, which can cross through the placenta into the foetus, and then can affect foetal development. Doctors and psychology biologists found the higher the level of cortisol in the mother's blood, the higher the level of cortisol in the amniotic fluid surrounding the foetus. Therefore, a higher level of stress hormone surrounds the growing baby. This hormone can then be absorbed into the baby and affect its development.

Average intermittent amounts of stress are okay between mother and child. But, daily stress, trauma, extreme depression and anxiety, and severe cases of abuse to the mother, unfortunately, can have a long-term effect on the child's brain development and future behaviour through the overproduction of cortisol.

The baby can be miscarried, born prematurely, have a low birth weight and of course, have mental health issues of its own.

These facts showed me that a person's mental health development starts in the womb, and I feel I must tell my story for the following reasons.

To bring further awareness that the mental health of a person starts in the womb before they are even born.

To bring further awareness, that the mother must not incur trauma or abuse of any kind.

To bring further awareness, even if a person does have suppressed anxieties, phobias or mental health issues, even way back in the womb, cognitively and spiritually there is hope to be free of the deep roots which keep you trapped.

And, getting back to Simon. I chose not to date him. I appreciated his honesty as he shared why his 21-year marriage ended. He had an affair. I couldn't move past the thought of repeating my history by being with someone who cheated. The risk was too high for me. Even though we parted ways I will be forever grateful for the significant healing process he instigated in my life. I am thankful now – for no more Band-Aids.

CHAPTER 32

Thank you for Saying Goodbye

The year was 2015. I hadn't heard from Laurie, my birth mother, for over ten years.

One night, Sarah and I were stalking Facebook for a snoop, as you do, and I found myself looking at Laurie's account. Sarah and I reminisced over our years with her, and I felt an intensity of gratitude flow into me for the mere fact she brought me into the world.

The feeling was so strong it brought me to tears, and I found myself talking to a picture of her on the screen. I shared my heart with her and thanked her for giving birth to me.

At 5.30 am the next morning, I woke up suddenly to a vision of Laurie's face hovering over me.

I heard her voice gently whisper in my ear, "Emma, please forgive me."

In my sleepiness, I replied, "Yes, Laurie, I forgive you."

Her face disappeared, and I drifted back to sleep, thinking I must be spiritually in tune with her since I spoke to her last night.

Two hours later at 7.30 am Laurie's sister, Aunty Lucy, phoned me to say Laurie had passed away exactly two hours ago from pancreatic cancer. She had been sick for a while.

I shared with Aunty Lucy the closeness I had with Laurie the night before and the encounter that morning with her asking for my forgiveness.

My visitation from her was a few minutes before she had died.

I can only assume Laurie knew she was about to leave this earth and was making things right in her heart with those around her.

Thank you, Laurie, for carrying me in your womb.
Thank you for being my birth mother.
Thank you for making things right with me.
Thank you for saying goodbye.

CHAPTER 33

Unfinished Business

I had forgiven Graham in my heart for the past, but there was no relationship between us. We didn't have a friendship, and I wouldn't even class him as an acquaintance. Yes, I had a brother when asked about my siblings, and if Mother asked him to do anything for me, he would, but other than a polite hello and goodbye, we shared nothing else.

We only saw each other at Christmas and family gatherings. Even though we passed each other like ships in the night, being near him still triggered my anxiety.

I had pushed my unresolved anguish between us down for so long all my life; there was no more room for me to push it down anymore. I was psychologically damaged. This condition can sometimes be called unfinished business.

All my life, everyone had ignored my unfinished business with Graham, and the use-by date for hiding my suppressed pain had reached its expiry date.

Graham's whole life dynamic had recently changed. Unfortunately, at 55 years of age, he went through a long and messy divorce. His two children had grown older and began to depend on him less. Dad had passed away. The family unit was now myself, Mother and Graham. I had no idea what his thoughts were or why now suddenly, he wanted to talk to me as if we have been best friends forever. For me, it was a shock.

We had gone out to dinner for a family celebration. Graham sat next to me and chatted away. Everyone in the restaurant assumed we were husband and wife. I politely put on my fake smile and melted into an internal panic attack. No one knew what was going on inside me. I had worn my mask of pretence all my life, and I did an excellent job of covering it up. Everyone was laughing and genuinely enjoying themselves – except me. The stress from that night turned into an anxiety episode that lasted for three weeks, and I was swept down into depression as well.

Enough was enough! I couldn't live bound in this emotional spiral anymore.

I was NOT going to wear my mask of people-pleasing anymore! I wasn't going to pretend something inside me wasn't happening when it was. NO MORE MASKS!

I would be true to myself, respect myself, and be honest.

Christmas was approaching. Just the thought of knowing I had to see Graham during this festive season set my anxiety off again. I had to tell Mother quite plainly; I couldn't do Christmas this year because I couldn't be near Graham anymore. No one in the family *EVER* skipped Christmas!

Mother was shocked at my out-of-the-blue statement and couldn't understand why. In all my attempts over the years to tell her about Graham and his violence, Mother never had a light bulb moment that the abuse was as bad and as frequent as it was.

But sharing with her again some of the cruel and tormenting assaults Graham had inflicted on me; she was listening with fresh ears and weeping sympathetically.

"Oh, my darling child, please forgive me for not realising how bad this was for you. I have failed you as a Mother, but we will make this right now."

I had no words of reply, just overwhelming gratitude. I was in my early 50's, and it had taken all these years for Mother to hear me.

Her tears were full of apology, regret, and failure. To me, they were a celebration – an acknowledgement I wanted for my life ever since I was a little girl. Mother insisted we call a meeting with Graham to discuss the situation and bring it out into the open and put it to rest.

She phoned Graham and confronted him with some of the abusive events I had shared with her. His response was, "Yeah, but that happened years ago." Mother replied firmly, "Yes, Graham, but the point here is, IT HAPPENED!"

Finally, justice was taking place.

I cannot begin to put into words how I felt. Hope flooded into every part of my being. For my mother to acknowledge this and stand next to me and say this abuse should never have happened, it wasn't okay then, and it's not okay now, was all I ever wanted.

The day of our intervention came. I was incredibly nervous. Although I fought hard never to feel like a victim in my life, this day, that's all I felt. But in the right way.

After approximately 50 years, Graham – was going to be held to account. Not on display in a courtroom, but a quiet family gathering.

I remember Mother telling me to be brave. I took a deep breath and pushed through my nerves. Here was my platform to share how I felt, then and now, for all the years Graham's abuse has affected me; how it has shaped me; how it has damaged me. As sad as it was – it was liberating.

I sat quietly in my chair reading from my long list of events I recalled that had damaged me.

Graham couldn't remember most of them although added a couple of instances he remembered that I had forgotten. He made a few comments to justify his actions in his defence. His attitude was neutral, with no hint of empathy. Just as well we were not in a court of law as his ego-based answers would not have held up his case. I knew Mother would have told him to say sorry, and he did what she asked. His apology had no heartfelt emotion, but it didn't matter. The truth was all out in the open. The abusive events which had occurred were exposed, and Graham was held accountable.

To be acknowledged for this grave, life-long wrong against me gave me incredible freedom.

The amount of healing I had within my spirit, soul, and body was immense. A new self-respect awoke inside me as the hidden closed door of injustice I had lived with all my life was now open. I could finally walk through it and be free. For the first time in my life, I carried a new power and dignity for the little girl inside and the woman I now was.

CHAPTER 34

Completely Healed

I planned a short trip to the Eastern States to visit my friends.

Sunday came, and I walked through the doors of the church looking forward to worshipping the Lord.

Everyone was welcoming and friendly. My friends hadn't come, but I was happy to sit by myself. The music started, and the songs were beautiful as they washed over the congregation.

Instantly, a wave of God's power fell upon me, and I sat down in my chair, put my head in my hands and sobbed. An older lady, in her late seventies, named Sylvia, was sitting behind me. She was a matriarch in the church and realising I was a visitor came and sat next to me with a box of tissues. Sylvia put her hand gently on my shoulder to let me know she was nearby for support.

She perceived God was healing my heart, so she sat silent.

Graham's face appeared in front of me. I wasn't quite sure why. It was a year since we had our intervention meeting, and I had moved on. But God knew there was still more to heal inside me.

A man stood up and brought forth a word from the Lord. His voice boomed across the room as if God himself was speaking. I can't exactly remember everything he said, but the essence was about forgiveness, letting go of hurts that happened when you were a child and God leading you here today for a specific deep healing. I knew it was God speaking personally to me. In that instant, I felt overwhelmed and loved by God, my Father.

Waves of God's love bathed me right to the core of my being. I whispered to Him, "Yes, of course, I forgive Graham." Overcome with emotion; I crumpled down in my chair. I had no physical strength in my body. The music kept playing, and the Holy Spirit kept washing over me; God was healing my soul.

I sat for the whole church service with my face buried in my hands. God's healing power washed over the years of past abuse from Graham. I hadn't known his injuries had scarred me this severely.

Another lady approached me. She didn't know anything about me as she spoke quietly in my ear. "God is showing me, Satan has been trying to destroy your life, since the moment of your conception in your mother's womb, BUT GOD, today, this day, breaks you free from that assignment."

She didn't know Laurie had tried to self-abort me with a knitting needle. "Yes," I said, "that word is right, and yes, ALL witchcraft spells and curses and generational bondages stop TODAY!"

Sylvia spent time with me during the week counselling me for inner healing, and the next four Sundays in the church service, God's Spirit washed over me powerfully, again and again, healing my soul.

My trauma was deep, layers deep, years deep, a life-time deep, generations deep. But now, I was COMPLETELY healed.

CHAPTER 35

Breath of Heaven

I am so glad I chose the narrow, dusty path, and because I did, God gave me many incredible life-changing encounters, experiences and healings.

God took all the damaged parts of my life and made me whole, even healing me right back to when I was in the womb.

It was on this narrow, dusty path; God showed me I must forgive those who hurt me and love them.

God showed me how to have a personal and intimate relationship with Jesus, that His word in the Bible is real, alive and powerful, and though I might not understand what is going on in my life, I can trust Him.

God gave me the strength to believe in myself and love who I am. He re-created the very fabric of my soul with His perfect, pure gold threads of love.

He sent his breath of heaven and healed my heart and mind from all the ingrained self-hate and gave me new eyes to see that I am His masterpiece.

I understand now Aunt Gretta's words are right: God makes everything beautiful – *in His way and in His time.*

As I continue on my journey through life, I have no fear of anything. I don't fear illness, tragedy, pain or even death itself. There is nothing that can happen to me that God and I cannot handle together.

I have faith, hope, and love, that has been tried and tested, and I know when I trust God, I will always have the VICTORY! For someone who feared *everything*, this is my miracle.

I might not know what my future holds – but I know WHO holds MY future – and I have peace. At any time, I have a place I can run to. It is in the palm of God's hand where I feel safe, secure and loved.

It is there I whisper to my Heavenly Father, "I love you; I will always love you; for I am, and always will be… *your child.*"

Dear reader, if you have identified with any part of my life or for more information on Mental Health, Spiritual Awakening, Trauma Healing and Wellness please visit *Heart Weaves* at www.meganreda.com for your FREE PDF workbook.

In my workbook you will find tools and Christian structured strategies for your own personal healing journey.

You can be free. You deserve to be free, and VICTORY is yours!

www.ingramcontent.com/pod-product-compliance
Lightning Source LLC
Chambersburg PA
CBHW040240010526
44107CB00065B/2818